The Potential for Health

KENNETH C. CALMAN
Chief Medical Officer
Whitehall, London, UK

Oxford New York Tokyo
OXFORD UNIVERSITY PRESS
1998

Oxford University Press, Great Clarendon Street, Oxford OX2 6DP

Oxford New York
Athens Auckland Bangkok Bogota Bombay
Buenos Aires Calcutta Cape Town Dar es Salaam
Delhi Florence Hong Kong Istanbul Karachi
Kuala Lumpur Madras Madrid Melbourne
Mexico City Nairobi Paris Singapore
Taipei Tokyo Toronto Warsaw
and associated companies in
Berlin Ibadan

Oxford is a trade mark of Oxford University Press

Published in the United States
by Oxford University Press Inc., New York

A catalogue record for this book is available from the British Library

Library of Congress Cataloging in Publication Data
Calman, Kenneth C. (Kenneth Charles)
Potential for health / Kenneth C. Calman
(Oxford medical publications)
Includes bibliographical references and index.
1. Health promotion. 2. Medical policy–United States. 3. Public health–United States. I. Title. II. Series.
RA395.A3C326 1998 362.1'0973–dc21 97-51536

ISBN 0 19 262585 3 (Hbk)
ISBN 0 19 262944 1 (Pbk)

Typeset by Downdell, Oxford
Printed in Great Britain by
Biddles Ltd, Guildford & King's Lynn

To Andrew, Lynn and Susan, who have kept me sane and made me laugh

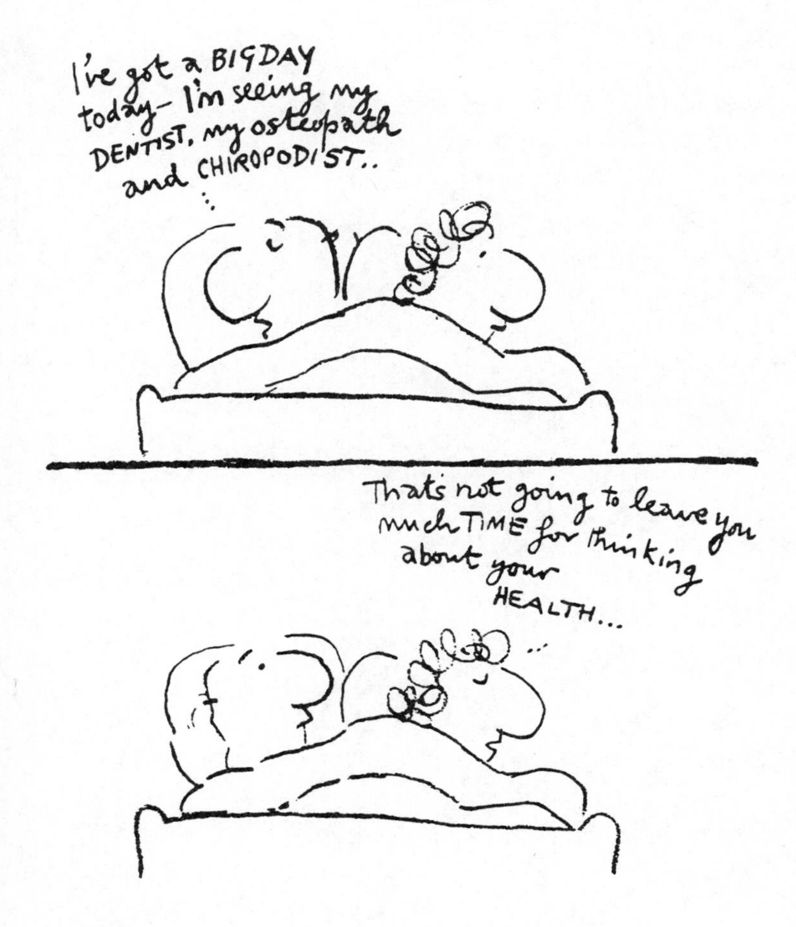

Preface

This book is the outcome of a series of talks, lectures, and speeches given to a wide variety of audiences over the last five or so years. It might be best described as a collection of essays, loosely woven together with the common thread of improving the health of the public. Taken together they represent a personal philosophy or point of view about health. The book is also, however, the product of considerable discussion and interaction between a variety of people—academics, clinicians, public, patients, and colleagues within the Department of Health and beyond. As some of my distinguished predecessors were prolific writers, there is therefore a precedent for this type of volume.

It is written for several different audiences but, generally, for a non-professional one. It is hoped that those sections which concentrate mainly on the medical role will be found interesting and relevant. For many professionals, some parts of the book will be very familiar, but I hope of some value. Finally, decision makers, in health policy and health care, may find this useful as a way of thinking about health matters.

In addition to health, the book covers issues such as management and education, which might initially be considered outside the remit. But they are key tools for change, and so are included. In a similar way, the discussion of medical education and medical values may be considered to be too narrow an approach. However, the lessons to be learned do have a wider context, and those in other professional groups may find them of value.

This book is not the end of the process, but a statement of where I am at the moment. Much may happen in the future to change the ideas and philosophy in this book, and I hope to be flexible enough to wish to modify my views accordingly as the knowledge base expands and research progresses.

While I have had considerable input from others regarding the thinking behind this book, in the final analysis it is my sole responsibility. It has, as its basis, the concept that health can be improved, using existing knowledge, and that the potential is there if only we could harness it.

London 1998 K. C. Calman

Contents

1 *Introduction, summary and conclusions* 1

1. Some basic issues 4
2. Historical aspects of health and health care 8
3. Factors influencing the outcome of health care 15
4. Target setting 17
5. Advancing knowledge 17
6. Public involvement in health and health care 18
7. Whose job is it to change health? 18
8. The ethical framework 19
9. A model for health and health care 20
10. Making it happen 26
11. Some conclusions 29

2 *Equity, poverty, and health for all* 30

1. The determinants of health 32
2. Equity, equality, and health for all 34
3. Poverty and health 39
4. Conclusions 44

3 *The health of the nation* 46

1. Key areas and targets 46
2. Delivering the strategy 48
3. The results so far 50
4. Our healthier nation 53

4 *Public and patient involvement in health and health care* 55

1. Introduction 55
2. Some general issues 56
3. Perceptions of health 59
4. Expectations of health and health care 64

5. Patient choice in health care 67
6. Public involvement in resource allocation and choices in health care 68
7. Risk communication 70
8. The role of the media in health 82
9. The public and their role in medical research and professional education 83
10. The public understanding of health, science, and medicine 85
11. Conclusions 85

5 Ethical issues in public health 87

1. Introduction 87
2. The ethical basis 88
3. The value base 89
4. Equity and equality 91
5. Some general issues 92
6. Some examples 93
7. Some conclusions 95

6 The humanities in clinical practice 97

1. Literature and medicine 98
2. Art and music in the hospital 101
3. The arts and the public 102
4. The humanities and clinical practice 103
5. The implications for managers 103

7 The medical detective 105

1. The role of intelligence in health and health care 105
2. Some examples of intelligence 108
3. The consequences of the intelligence function 109
4. The role of patients and the public 112
5. Some conclusions 112

8 The science and art of public health 114

1. The science of public health 114
2. The art of public health 118
3. The potential of research affecting the socio-economic approach to prevention 127
4. Research 131
5. Some final thoughts 136
6. A postscript on hygiene 136

9 *International aspects of health* 138

1. Introduction 138
2. The impact of international aspects of health 138
3. Some current health problems 139
4. Health in Europe 140
5. Factors influencing international variations in the levels of health 142
6. Health for all 145
7. Ethical issues in international health 145
8. Partnerships in health 148
9. Summary 148

10 *Health care* 150

1. What is health care? 150
2. Quality of life 151
3. Quality of care 154
4. Outcomes and effectiveness 159
5. Evidence-based medicine 162
6. Clinical audit 164
7. Maintaining professional standards: the role of mentoring 168
8. Management and health services 169
9. Making choices: issues of resource allocation 173
10. Information technology 177
11. Communication 178
12. Tales and legends in clinical practice 182
13. Memories: a neglected concept in care 185

11 *Some special issues in health care* 189

1. Introduction 189
2. Primary care 189
3. Mental health 190
4. The elderly 191
5. Adolescence 192
6. The health of men 193
7. The health of women and the role of women in health 193
8. Disability 194
9. Rehabilitation 195
10. Health in the workplace 196
11. Conclusions 196

12 Professional issues 197

1. Introduction 197
2. The profession of medicine 198
3. The future of specialization in medicine 207
4. Do we need a new Hippocratic Oath? 216
5. Professional education 224
6. Working together: teamwork 237

13 Looking to the future: some big issues ahead 243

1. Introduction 243
2. Social and economic factors 243
3. Understanding disease 246
4. Clinical practice 247
5. Public health issues 249
6. Some conclusions 251

14 Making it happen 252

1. Introduction 252
2. Change at different levels 255
3. Leadership 260
4. The future 261

15 Envoi 263

Index 269

1

Introduction, summary and conclusions

***'Where there is no vision the people perish'* Proverbs**

This book has two purposes. First to identify key issues in health and health care, and second to identify ways in which improvements in both might occur. Its title, 'The potential for health', recognizes that more might be achieved *now* to improve health, health care, and quality of life, if we were able to use our existing knowledge more effectively. That potential can be realized. It is also acknowledged that change will only occur through people —whether they are the public at large, patients, politicians or decision makers, or health professionals. The book will only be of value if it stimulates discussion and argument.

Before developing these themes further it is relevant to consider in more detail the use of the word 'potential'. The main reason for choosing this word was a recognition that improving health was 'possible but not yet actual' (to use the dictionary definition) and that much more could be achieved. But the word has other connotations:

1. Potential is associated with the concept of energy—the capacity to do work—if the energy can be harnessed. The waterfall provides a clear visual analogy as to the power of potential energy. Releasing the power is the key.
2. Potential also implies the ability to transform or change from one form of energy into another. This is crucial as one of the key elements implied in the process of change

is the transformation and empowerment of people to improve their own health and that of others.

3. Potential also signifies a gap between what is now, and what could be. It is the narrowing of the gap which provides the impetus for this book.

But the most obvious question which might be raised at this stage is 'What's in it for me?'. What would the benefits be for me, for my organization, or group, if I put some energy into initiating change? Will it mean giving up the things I enjoy? Will it actually reduce the quality of life? Do I really want to live longer and be miserable? Politically will it take me into difficult areas? What will it mean for my professional role? What will the costs be to my organization? These are clearly uncomfortable questions, and difficult ones to answer—but they need to be tackled. People or organizations are unlikely to change, or even wish to change, unless the benefits can be made visible and the perception of the benefits is real. That is the challenge, central to which will be the theme of quality of life, of fun, and enjoyment. Being healthy is a positive concept and should be valued.

Seven very general principles can be highlighted at the outset which set the tone for the rest of the book:

1. The overall objective is to improve health, health care, and quality of life. This latter aspect is crucial and will be referred to throughout the book. The aim is to make people feel better and enjoy life in addition to living longer. Being healthy is a good thing to be, and should not be associated with negative images of what not to do.

2. It needs to be recognized that the objective of being healthy concerns the whole population and is about health for all. This phrase 'health for all' is not just rhetoric but implies a need to ensure that all sections of the population—whoever they are, wherever they live, whatever they do or believe—are part of the process. Everyone should have the opportunity to realise his or her 'potential for health' regardless of race, social class, geography, and so

on. The debate however is moving on and perhaps a more useful phrase is 'health *by* all', indicating the need for involvement and ownership of health. Thus the importance of equity in improving health is emphasized right from the start of this book. To achieve this there is a need to set out a national strategy to improve health.

3. The whole purpose is to focus resources, enthusiasm, energy, and skills on people—not to please doctors, nurses, decision makers, or anyone else. The aim of being healthy is for the benefit of the public and needs to involve a wide range of sectors including environment, education, social services, and employment. The involvement of patients and the public in the process is essential; indeed the support and encouragement of self-care constitutes a great proportion of health service resources and needs to be recognized.

4. An intelligence or surveillance system is required to ensure that changes in health and in the outcome of health care are identified early and acted upon, and that there is an effective monitoring system in place to document such changes.

5. From the point of view of health care it is necessary to ensure that decisions are made on the basis of evidence and on the outcomes to be achieved. Only when this scientific approach and the importance of the knowledge base has pervaded the service will it be possible to make rational decisions about care. We need more information about what determines health and quality of health care. An understanding of these determinants and influences is very important.

6. The basis of change is education, built on a knowledge base which is continually revised and updated by research. Education and research remain the foundations of change.

7. Ethical and moral issues are at the heart of the process of change and provide the framework around which decisions

are made. The values which are held by those involved in health and health care are crucial and determine the nature of the services provided and the approach to improving health.

The remainder of this chapter will set out the broad issues and come to some general conclusions as to how health might be improved. It summarizes much of the discussion presented throughout the book and the conclusions which are developed more fully in Chapter 14. It also deals with some historical aspects of health and health care, and sets out a model of health which synthesizes the thinking in the book.

This chapter is then followed by a series of chapters on public health matters including health for all, a healthier nation, patient and public partnerships, ethical issues, the art and science of public health, and international issues. There are then sections on health care and professional issues. Concluding chapters are about looking to the future and making it happen, with a final personal envoi. These chapters expand on this introductory chapter.

1. Some basic issues

The definition of health

So far it has been assumed that we know what is meant by health and that the purpose of 'being healthy' is clear. The World Health Organisation's definition of health is a good starting point, but not the only one. The definition states that 'health is a state of complete physical and mental well-being and not merely the absence of disease or infirmity'. Several issues follow from this definition. First, that health is a relative term and cannot be regarded as an absolute, in that it can always be improved. This is one of the major assumptions in this book. Second, there are both positive and negative aspects of health. Feeling well and being ill are both parts of the same concept.

Finally, health should be considered in an holistic way, in that many factors are relevant—physical, emotional and spiritual, psychological, social, and intellectual. (The Pepsi concept.)

Determinants of health

If the definition given is accepted for the moment, it is possible to begin to outline those factors which influence health. (Factors influencing health care will be discussed in a subsequent section in this chapter.) Such factors include:

1. *Genetic factors*: these are of considerable importance to our understanding and management of health and disease. As more and more genes are recognized which have an impact on health, so the implications of this will be apparent. For example, the screening of individuals and populations will become increasingly possible, bringing with it a range of ethical and moral issues, in addition to clinical ones.

2. *The environment*: this includes all those elements in the external world which might have an impact on health, such as the quality of air, water, and soil, and exposure to radiation and communicable disease. This factor is closely related to 'Agenda 21'— a strategy developed by the United Nations to link the environment with a variety of issues including health and sustainable development.

3. *Lifestyle*: many aspects of how we live and behave affect our health. Dietary habits, smoking, drugs, alcohol, and sexual behaviour are all part of this.

4. *Social and economic factors*: it is well recorded that these factors influence health in many ways. For example, different cultural backgrounds, employment status, income, housing, and social class are all relevant. Education, and the opportunities it presents, is also an important part of this.

5. *Health services*: the provision of a health care service contributes to health by in some instances curing the individual, in others reducing disability, or improving quality of life.

It is likely that in the development of any specific disease, several of these factors will be relevant. For example, in diabetes there is both a genetic and lifestyle component, and an important contribution from the health service. In coronary heart disease, genetic factors, lifestyle, social and economic factors, and the health service are all relevant. Taking tuberculosis as a final example, the environment, lifestyle, social and economic factors, and the health service are all important. There will be a different emphasis on each of the factors mentioned for these diseases. In association with those factors which influence health care, these issues can be brought together into a model for health.

It should also be clear that if the health of a population is to be improved then the least effective way to achieve this, overall, is through health services. The other four factors are considered to be more important. This issue will be developed later in the book.

Quality of life and the purpose of health

Quality of life is a concept which is generally understood, but is very difficult to define. Essentially it relates to the gap between what an individual or community want and what is available to them, to the differences between dreams and aspirations and the reality. It is clearly subjective and linked to past experiences, future hopes, and the culture of the group or the community. No matter how difficult it is to define quality of life, it should be the end point by which health programmes are judged. It should cover all aspects of life—physical health being only one of a whole range of issues (physical, emotional, psychological, social, and spiritual) which can affect or influence the quality of life. People who are ill or disabled can be happy; people who are physically well may not be. Quality of life is therefore the summation of many factors synthesized to give an overall feeling of well-being.

This in turn raises an important issue concerning the purpose of health. Is health a means of obtaining a better quality of life, or is health and being healthy an end in itself? The answer to the question is fundamental. If health is an end in itself then resources, skills, and expertise should be directed at maintaining the highest levels of health for the individual and the population, sometimes to the exclusion of other issues which might improve quality of life. If on the other hand health is one means of improving quality of life then it becomes evident that other dimensions of life need to be supported. Populations and groups therefore need to consider carefully the level of health which is sustainable for their community and relate this to the level of resources available. For the purposes of this book it will be assumed that health is a means by which quality of life can be improved, but that other aspects of life such as education, housing, the environment, transport, law and security are also important, both to individuals and to society as a whole. For a fuller discussion of this see Daniel Callaghan's book, *What kind of life*.

Related to this is the question as to why we should improve health at all, if all we achieve is a longer lifespan with increasing disability. This of course is not the objective. What is required is a programme of action which prolongs life but at the same time reduces morbidity to a minimum. This 'compression of morbidity' to the shortest length of time is important. It is about adding 'life to years' as well as 'years to life'.

Throughout this book the potential conflict between the needs and expectations of individuals and communities and the variations in health and health care which exist will be repeatedly examined. If the purpose of health and health care is to keep everyone healthy then resources would be exhausted rapidly. Within finite resources, no matter what the level, this would occur. The rights of the individual to full health and access to all available health care may conflict with the needs of the community as a whole. This issue needs to be debated fully and is discussed in more detail in subsequent chapters. Equity is a key principle in improving the potential for health.

'The health of the people is really the foundation upon which all their powers of state depend.' This remark by Disraeli poses a further question—what is the vision for the *nation's* health to be? It must be to achieve an overall improvement in the nation's health which, in turn, will improve the quality of life for the individual and the community. This aim is:

(1) holistic, in that it covers physical, psychological, social, and spiritual aspects of life; it puts the patient and the community first;
(2) ecological, in that it puts human health in the context of the world as a whole, and relates human activity to animal and plant life, and the wider environment;
(3) intersectoral, in that it acknowledges that a wide range of agencies and individuals need to be involved in achieving the potential.
(4) equitable, in that it recognizes that the variations in health which exist must be tackled.

The aim is concerned both with positive health and with improving the outcome of health care. It requires, at its foundation, better ways of measuring and monitoring the nation's health over time.

2. Historical aspects of health and health care

This section cannot be considered as a proper 'history' of health and health care. It sets out however some personal reflections on the changes which have occurred, particularly over the last two hundred years, and uses them to highlight some relevant issues. It illustrates where we have come from, how much of the potential we have realized, and what have been the driving forces and mechanisms of change. In this context it should be seen as a scene setting exercise for the rest of the book.

As will be illustrated, many of the changes which have occurred have had to wait, first on rational explanation (for example, the discovery of the bacterial origin of disease) and secondly, on those of authority recognizing the issue and tackling it. In public health terms the recognition of the value of taking action to improve health has been clear since biblical times. Hippocrates had also appreciated the importance of public health matters and in his writing on 'airs, waters and places' noted the importance of such factors in the determination of health. Indeed, he encouraged the physician to ask questions about such matters in the making of the diagnosis. It is interesting to note that the introduction of quarantine in medieval Italy and France, the use of cowpox vaccination, the importance of vitamin C, the role of adequate housing, and the problem of overcrowding all preceded the definitive knowledge of the science and the full explanation of the link between the preventative measure and the disease.

The nineteenth century

The explosion of interest in public health began in the middle of the nineteenth century with the movement for sanitary reform and the beginning of voluntary and poor law hospital provision. From then on a need for medical or scientific explanations for change, based on evidence, became increasingly important. For an interesting example of the problems faced by some cities and the lessons which can be learned, the book *Death in Hamburg. Society and politics in the cholera years 1830–1910* by Richard J. Evans provides fascinating insights. During the nineteenth century however, changes in social conditions, including housing, began to have an impact and measures of health, such as morbidity rates and maternal and infant mortality, began to alter. There was increasing interest in the workplace and the dangers and hazards associated with some occupations.

One of the most interesting aspects of this time was the recognition of the importance of collection and analysis of information. Who died of what, and where? Were there any patterns or linking factors? Why did one place do better or worse than another? While information in the form of 'Bills of Mortality' had been available in many parts of the country, the systematic collection of data did not occur routinely. Nowadays, it is perhaps difficult to appreciate just how important data collection and analysis was. Yet the mechanisms set up then to gather information still provide the basis of the monitoring and surveillance systems we have at present. The intelligence networks established were powerful factors, for example, in the control of infectious disease. It should also be recognized just what the impact of such figures was on decision makers. Faced with carefully collected data showing the extent of the disease in a particular place, and with methods of reducing the illness available, it was difficult not to act. For those practising public health at present, this lesson should not be lost.

The changes in health which resulted were pursued by legislation and set standards of building, sanitation, control of infectious disease, and safety in the workplace—all subjects which go beyond the health service. Looking back it becomes clear what a remarkable impact such changes have had on health. Changes in health and safety in the workplace deserve special mention. Working conditions, the age of starting work, the identification of specific industrial diseases are issues that have all been confronted, and continue to be so as new hazards appear. The potential to improve health in this one area has been tackled head on, though much still remains to be done.

Infant mortality began to change and with it the family size. (A visit to any graveyard with nineteenth-century headstones provides a dramatic and visual account of the loss to society of infants, children, and young people.) During the nineteenth century, two other major factors began to influence health. The first was education. Standards began to rise and,as a determinant of health, an educated population is one of the most crucial. The second was the greater economic prosperity of the country during the latter part of the century. Economic prosperity and health care are closely related—an association still relevant today.

Again, during the latter part of the nineteenth century two major scientific advances were to change the course of medical care: anaesthesia and antisepsis. It began to be possible to operate on patients with some safety and with remarkable success. Medical treatment at this time was limited to a few effective drugs and diagnosis was essentially clinical, without the benefits of X-rays and laboratory analysis. Immunization at last had a rational base and there was an expansion in the number of infectious diseases against which effective vaccines became available. Vaccination remains one of the most powerful methods of prevention of disease, and amongst the most cost effective.

The twentieth century

By the beginning of the twentieth century there was a much greater understanding of disease. Pathology as a specialty had arrived and with it bacteriology, and this scientific base was beginning to make rational intervention more feasible. Diagnosis became clearer and it became possible to set out the prognosis of disease, determine its natural history, and understand the factors which influenced recovery. The discovery of X-rays assisted in this process. The classification of disease changed and allowed a more structured approach to diagnosis. A rather more general point can be made here about the diagnosis and classification of disease. Almost every major advance in medicine has been associated with a change in the way in which disease is categorized. Indeed it could be said that the history of medicine is about the reclassification of disease. Looking ahead to the changes which will come about by a greater understanding of genetic influences on health, the same is likely to be the case.

More medical treatments became available in the early twentieth century and the first antibiotics showed the enormous potential which would be realized later in the century.

The discovery of insulin and other hormones, vitamins, and new drugs to help treat heart disease and lung disease seemed to indicate during the first half of the century that with a few more research breakthroughs, all the problems would be solved.

There were also major social and economic changes during this time, building on the work of the earlier pioneers. One of the most important was the changing role of women—a factor of central importance to improving health. Their right to vote and take part in decision making was fundamental to change. Housing conditions had improved, although the problems of overcrowding and slums were still apparent.

In the first half of the twentieth century there was considerable movement and expansion of the population, with growth occurring mainly in the large towns. 'Urbanization' has since become a feature of all countries in the world, with some cities reaching 'mega proportions' with population sizes of 20 to 30 million. This explosion of population and migration increased the chances of spread of infection and in some places put an intolerable strain on water and sanitation. The great pioneering works on safe and reliable sources of water and removal of sewage began at this time. The recognition that environmental factors were important in improving health also became evident.

The next great watershed was the Second World War. It demonstrated the value of new surgical techniques, the use of blood transfusion, antibiotics, and in particular anti-tuberculous therapy. It was during this time that the great experiment in social engineering—the National Health Service—was conceived and subsequently born in 1948. The National Health Service has been a remarkable success and the envy of the world. The fact that all citizens have access to health care, free at the point of delivery, has been a significant factor in improving health. The quality of medical care in this country is of the highest order, and compares with any in the world. Particular mention should be made of general practice and primary care. Every person has a right to have a general practitioner and from this the ability to deliver improved health through vaccination, health promotion, early diagnosis, and treatment has become a reality unmatched in any other country. The quality of general practice and primary care is outstanding and is the bedrock of the whole health care system.

This current period, the second half of the twentieth century, has also seen the most remarkable developments in medical care and diagnosis. The treatment of some forms of cancer and heart disease, transplantation of organs, joint replacement, new diagnostic techniques such as CT scanning and MRI imaging have all had a major effect. The impact of molecular biology and genetics in public health and health care is just at the threshold. Such a short list can only briefly describe the huge changes which have occurred. Life-saving procedures and improving the quality of life of individuals are commonplace and there is, to some extent, a feeling that medical science can do anything. To those on the inside, this has never been the case. The limits to medical care are clear which is why to realize the potential of health requires more than just advances in medical science. It needs to take into account developments in science, sociology, and medicine and use them to improve health across a wide range of areas—education, transport, environment, food safety, and so on—by developing policies reflecting the knowledge available.

In the latter part of the nineteenth century there were important moves to improve the education of doctors, and the General Medical Council was established to provide assurance to the public of the quality of medical education. The second part of the twentieth century has also seen some important developments in educational methods, competency assessment, and continuing education. Other professional groups have been equally active and there is a general recognition, based on generations of experience, that an educated professional workforce is essential to the delivery of quality care. During the second part of the twentieth century, public health advances have not been forgotten: the significant health effects of cigarette smoking were recognized; environmental issues were also seen to be important; and, together, the remarkable effects of the Clean Air Act on improving the quality of air, seat-belt legislation, drink driving campaigns, breast feeding initiatives, and childhood immunization rates of over 95 per cent, have all contributed to a steady lowering of mortality and morbidity.

However, the development of the NHS, the importance of good quality health care, and rapid advances in medical practice only seem to emphasize two things. The first relates to unmet need and the finite nature of resources. The second, to the increasing realization that medical advance, on its own, would not be sufficient to improve the health of the population. Medicine and science could lead, could identify changes required, and could point the way forward—but more was needed. Social and economic factors together with personal lifestyle changes must also be considered.

The first issue raises the fact that as medical science has advanced in terms of diagnosis and treatment, with the ability to improve lifespan and quality of life, it becomes clearer that it may never be possible to meet needs within finite resources. This is not a new dilemma, but it has become increasingly evident and has begun to focus attention on the current great revolution in medical education and medical care—the importance of defining the outcomes of care, and the effectiveness of treatment. It raises questions of rationing and priority setting. The second issue relates to the importance of non-medical factors in improving health, and some practical examples may help to illustrate this. The first evidence that cigarette smoking was harmful to health came in the 1930s and by the 1960s it was well established. The signs were clear but at a population, and a personal level, decisions to stop smoking are still not being made. Similarly with HIV infection, medical science has clearly identified the mode of spread of the infection as being related to unprotected sexual intercourse or by the transfer of infected blood. Yet the spread continues. What is required, in some instances therefore, is not more evidence, but a change in attitude and behaviour.

From this very brief review, the lessons of the past could perhaps include:

- the importance of quality of life, not just longevity
- the need for a knowledge base in medicine and science
- the importance of social and economic factors
- the need for environmental factors to be considered
- the central role of education
- the role of women
- the importance of our health service being based in primary care
- the need for resource allocations to be based on outcomes and effectiveness.

Today, some of these issues, learned in the hard school of experience, may need to be learned again. If the potential for health is to be realized, each of these require to be recognized. This list of factors will be referred to throughout the book.

3. Factors influencing the outcome of health care

To develop a strategy for improving health also requires an understanding of the factors that influence health care outcomes. Factors determining health have already been defined as biological and genetic, environmental, lifestyle, social and economic, and health services. Health care is that part of influencing or improving health which requires advice, a service (including prevention and early diagnosis), treatment, or care to be provided by an individual (self-care) or the community in the form of family or friends, a voluntary organization, or a health care professional. In most instances care is provided by someone who is not a health care professional and, most frequently, by a woman. In many cultures the 'wise woman' of the village or town provides most of the health advice.

A health care outcome is the result of one or more episodes of care (including treatment) provided over a period of time, for an individual or community. Outcomes are related to the objectives of care set by the patient and staff at the start of the episode. As with the determinants of health, there are five factors which can be considered as affecting the outcome of health care:

(1) Health status of the individual and community. The health status in terms of fitness or the presence of associated diseases is clearly relevant at the time of diagnosis and the start of treatment or care.
(2) The disease, its natural history, stage at diagnosis, and prognosis. This may well be the most important determinant. The difference between the outcome in lung cancer and the common cold is obvious, but even within disease categories there may be substantial differences in outcome.
(3) Treatment, including rehabilitation and its effectiveness. For some illnesses the treatment is very effective, even curative, and may be the major determinant of the outcome. For others this is currently not the case.
(4) The skill mix of those providing the care. Educational and professional skills and expertise are clearly relevant.
(5) Facilities and resources to provide health care. This should not be seen only in financial terms, but should also relate to skills, expertise, and equipment.

In each of these areas there is a clear need for more information and research. Indeed, one of the purposes of listing such factors is that they highlight, in individual diseases, where further work is required. They also illustrate the close relationship between health and its determinants, and those factors which influence health care outcomes. There are clear areas of overlap.

A further point in listing these factors is that it becomes very clear that the issues raised are very complex, involve a wide range of agencies, and necessitate a multidisciplinary response, from basic science to sociology. The list of determinants also focuses attention on those who have a responsibility to improve health—individuals, the community, professionals, the public voluntary and private sectors, the faith communities, and politicians. The international nature of health problems also becomes clear when these factors are reviewed.

4. Target setting

Setting targets for improving health and health care is one way in which direction can be set, resources identified, the magnitude of the task identified, and progress monitored. They assist in the communication of the objectives and the mechanisms to achieve them. They can encourage commitment from the key players and allow everyone to pull in the same direction. Targets may need local interpretation to ensure local ownership, and their disadvantage is that if they are not reached then blame may be placed on one party or another. This is to misunderstand the nature of targets, particularly in relation to health, where a host of factors may make their achievement more difficult, or in some cases, easier. Thus, a target set for the reduction in the mortality of coronary heart disease over a 10-year period might change significantly if a new treatment became available which effectively reduced the death rate. All targets should be reviewed regularly.

5. Advancing knowledge

A very important part of the professional contribution to changing health has been the advances made in knowledge, both in health and health care. The importance of the curiosity motive and the research base must be stressed. The contributions from other disciplines need to be recognized, and this includes sociology, psychology, economics, geography, the basic sciences, and, from the point of view of the caring aspects of health care, the arts and the humanities and the faith communities. This knowledge base is very important but, in the management of uncertainty and in communicating with patients, the 'Art of Medicine' must not be forgotten.

The improvement of health care outcomes (survival rate, quality of life, and so on) has been driven by medical and other professional staff developing better methods of treatment and care. The challenge is to ensure that these new methods are rapidly introduced across the population as a whole. Such implementation needs to be backed up by evaluation and clinical audit.

6. Public involvement in health and health care

A major theme in this book is the need for increasing involvement of patients and the public in health and health care. The public's perception of health, health beliefs, and of social and cultural aspects of personal and community life are well recognized and important to changing health. The environment in which people live and work has a major impact on health, as do cultural and social conditions. The environment can also affect the level of involvement in health-related matters. There are groups who feel isolated and alienated and not part of the community as a whole. Thus, while the need to involve patients and the public in improving health is paramount, the barriers to doing so need to be appreciated. We have to bring such communities back into society.

7. Whose job is it to change health?

The short answer to this question is 'everybodys'. The public have an important role to play: the need for community involvement has already been mentioned, and there are many good examples where the community, often the women, have decided that enough is enough and that things need to change. The concept of the healthy city, village, school, or hospital focuses such energy. Patients also need to be involved. They have great experiences of illness, they know what the problems are, and they can use this to help others. Professionals need to respond to this potential and to work with patients to improve the health care of others. There is a strong wish to do so, and it should not be stifled or the messages not heard. The role of community health councils and the voluntary sector is also important.

Professionals have a major role in improving health and health care. They can do this by:

- providing a high standard of care
- maintaining and monitoring these standards over the years
- listening to patients and the public
- carrying out research to understand disease and improve treatment
- working with other professionals to improve care
- considering ethical implications of health and health care
- managing and using resources wisely.

These will be discussed further in Chapter 12.

Politicians and other decision makers also have a most important role. They look at the wider issues which affect health from across all government departments: policies in such as the environment, transport, economics, employment, and housing all have an impact. Thus the health implications of policy need to be checked on each occasion that changes are made. This is a unique function of government, and as the 'Our Healthier Nation' policy in England demonstrates, the co-ordination of health initiatives across government has great value.

Finally, as was mentioned on page 3, the key to unlocking the potential is health *by* all. We all have both a personal and a social responsibility to improve health. The contributions of the individual for his or her own work and those with whom they are in contact, is part of this.

8. The ethical framework

At the foundation of all this is an ethical framework or value base. In almost all aspects of health, choices have to be made about resources, treatments, priorities, the environment, research, and so on. Equity is at the heart of this. Ethical decisions are generally made on the basis of a set of values, the determination of which helps understanding of how such decisions are made. Such an ethical framework will be a thread throughout this book.

9. A model for health and health care

Introduction

Reference has been made on several occasions in this chapter for the need to develop models of health and health care. To understand the basis of improving health it is useful to have a framework or model to assist in making decisions and setting priorities. Models are useful for several reasons:

- they assist in the interpretation of health data
- they can be used to predict outcome
- they can be used to identify areas of action
- they can determine informational, research, and educational needs.

Any model that is developed must be relevant both to the individual and the community and, as real life is likely to be so complex and multifactorial, the model must represent a gross simplification of the actual situation. However, even the development of a crude model might help to communicate some sense of the issues involved and illuminate the potential for change. The model developed here is thus presented as an aid to communication. Such models also provide the framework within which health issues can be debated and the strategic intent made more explicit. Models and frameworks should therefore clarify the purpose and vision, and ensure that the long-term objectives are kept in focus. This is particularly the case with health issues where the time-scale for change may be measured in years or decades.

The development of the strategy is, in itself, not sufficient. What is also required, and which flows from the strategy, is an action plan which sets out the objectives, has strong top management and political support, and which has the necessary resources, skills, and expertise to make it happen. Carl von Clausewitz, a Prussian soldier, in his book *On war*, puts it very clearly. To win a war, he says, requires full political support, a strategy with clear objectives, commanders in the field to take tactical and operational decisions, and an effective supply line for logistic support, food, ammunition, and so on. So it is with health, and if any of the components are absent full success cannot be achieved.

Two targets to aim for

It is possible to combine the determinants of health and those factors which influence health outcomes into a model which can be used to assist decision making and setting priorities. Using the model, a strategy and action plan to improve health can be more easily defined and regularly updated and evaluated. The two targets are improved health and health care.

The basic model consists of integrating the determinants of health and outcomes of health care, already described, and linking these with methods of assessing the outcome of any intervention. Such assessment measures might range from improved health, reduction in mortality or disability, recovery from illness, or a change in quality of life. The determinants and influencing factors may also be modified. Thus the health determinants can be influenced by measures to promote or protect health, prevent illness, and encourage the active involvement of the public and other key partners. In a similar way those factors which influence health care can themselves be modified by early diagnosis and screening, rehabilitation, the role of carers, patient involvement, and the interaction with other groups and organizations such as local authorities and voluntary agencies.

Added to this basic model are research and education, which have an important influence on outcomes. Ethical issues provide a broad and overarching framework within which the model operates, reflecting the importance of values. The model can be further refined by the consideration of information, intelligence and surveillance, and methods to predict health.

Finally, external factors such as national, European, or global issues (for example, climate change) may also be relevant. The model can be represented both diagrammatically and in tabular form, as shown in Fig. 1.1 and Table 1.1.

Using the model

To use the model, first identify a topic, which might be a disease or a risk factor, then consider which particular

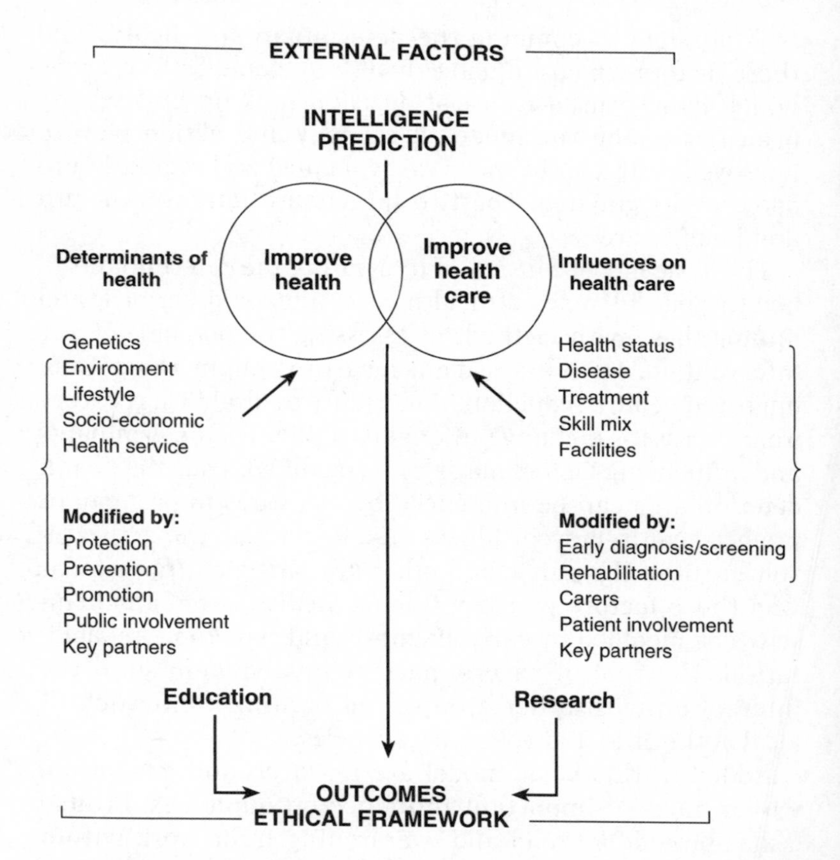

Fig. 1.1—A model for health and health care—the two targets.

Table 1.1—A model for health.

Topic: Risk factor, disease
Group: Individual, population
Special group: Maternity, children, adolescents, elderly, adult, mental health, etc.

Diagnosis/risk factor		Comment	Responsibility and action
Health	Genetic		
	Environmental		
	Lifestyle		
	Socio-economic		
Modified by	Protection		
	Promotion		
	Prevention		
	Public involvement		
	Key partners		
Health care	Patient		
	Disease		
	Treatment		
	Skills		
	Facilities		
Modified by	Early diagnosis		
	Emergency		
	Rehabilitation		
	Patient involvement		
	Carers		
	Key partners		
General	Research		
	Education		
	Intelligence		
	Prediction		
Outcome measures			
Ethical issues			
External factors			

Priorities identified	Action
1.	1.
2.	2.
3.	3.

patient or population group is to be investigated. In a systematic way, using Table 1.1, review each of the components, recording the information available and its possible impact on the outcome. It is important to note where evidence is not available or where gaps in knowledge occur, as this will identify areas for research. Finally, the whole model is considered and priorities and actions identified which are both practical and lead to improvement in health or the outcome of health care. Some examples may help to illustrate this more effectively. They are presented for discussion only and there is scope for debate about the conclusions. That is the purpose of the process.

Example 1: dementia The subject needs careful definition as several forms of disease fall into this category. The population is generally elderly, but some important dementias occur in younger groups, for example, CJD. This might be considered separately. In the 'health box', genetic factors may be relevant, but the others do not seem to be so. In the 'modifying box', health promotion probably has little place, though it is clear that public involvement and understanding are crucial. Under 'health care', the major issues are the progression of disease, lack of effectiveness of treatment, the importance of trained staff, and the role of carers. There is a clear need for more epidemiological data and more research is required.
Priorities identified: need for staff training, carer support, more research.

Example 2: lung cancer There is little genetic influence and the main factor in its causation is cigarette smoking. This is more obvious in lower social classes. Health promotion and smoking cessation are relevant. As a disease it is very difficult to treat, and there are no effective screening techniques.
Priorities identified: co-ordinated approach to smoking control including advertising and price controls. More research on prevention (behavioural modification), treatment, and smoking cessation.

Example 3: childhood accidents The environment, lifestyle of parents, and social factors are all relevant. Health promotion and public involvement are central. Treatment is generally good and there needs to be an emphasis on rehabilitation. **Priorities identified: social and economic factors, play areas, local involvement, and community development projects.**

Some conclusions

The model is relatively simple to operate, but there is no substitute for an in-depth study of each topic. The model can be used by a variety of groups such as patients, professionals, managers, and politicians, each of which is likely to identify different priorities. This can be useful in bringing out the differences in approach and in understanding the process of improving health.

Experience across the world has shown that to improve health an integrated and strategic long-term approach is required. In general, a limited number of topics are chosen to reflect major determinants of health and the burden of disease. Targets are set and a wide variety of groups and organizations from all sectors are involved in the process of change. There should be a regular process of monitoring and evaluation.

The root causes of ill health such as poverty, social conditions, employment, housing, transport, environmental pollution, and education need a national focus. Community development projects at local level allow full public involvement and complete deployment of all the local resources in the statutory and voluntary sectors. Individuals and families also need to recognize that they too have a responsibility to maintain and improve their health. Professionals should see their role in a different light, being concerned not only with treating illness but in improving the health of those with whom they come into contact.

There are major inequalities in health in this country. Almost every investigation into every disease shows this. Many, though not all, are avoidable. To tackle these differences will require commitment, skills, and expertise. The knowledge is available and the potential can be realized if we have the courage and leadership to drive the changes through.

10. Making it happen

The purpose of the process described so far is to improve health and health care for individuals and the population as a whole and to outline those factors which influence and determine the outcome. How can we make it happen? This subject is dealt with in detail in Chapter 14, but is summarized here for completeness.

There are two important considerations to be discussed before going into detail about the steps to be taken. The first of these is that the basis for 'making it happen' is similar to that of education—a process that chiefly aims to change behaviour. One of the fundamental principles of learning is to begin with what the learner already knows, and to build on it. We need to begin where people are at, and not where we think they are. Listening to them is crucial. The second consideration is that existing knowledge about improving health already provides the means to change, and while it will always be useful to have more evidence, getting started is important. New knowledge will always be 'just around the corner', but there should be no delay in beginning.

Releasing the potential will always be through people, using their enormous capacity to think creatively and positively. We need to harness that brain power and energy. A wide range of people are involved—from individuals, professionals, the public, communities, to organizations and politicians.

The personal level This is the most difficult of all, and raises a number of personal questions such as 'Is it worth it?' 'Will the pain be worth the gain?'. There are a few measures which, if considered seriously, can help to improve health. Whilst it is not possible to say in any individual how effective they might be, here are 10 things worth thinking about.

Unlike the ten commandments, not every statement need be attempted:

1. Enjoy life. Being healthy is a good thing to be.
2. Take regular, moderate exercise consistent with your age and medical condition.
3. Enjoy your food. Eat a balanced diet, and keep you weight under control.
4. Feeling good about yourself is not easy, but important. Stress is common; make sure you have some quiet time on your own.
5. Sexual health is also important. Practise safe sex.
6. Think about the health of your family and friends. Being a good parent would be part of this.
7. Look after yourself if you have an illness. Make sure you see your doctor if you are concerned.
8. Enjoy the sunshine but take precautions by wearing appropriate clothes and sunscreens.
9. Accidents and injuries can be prevented. Do a regular 'accident check' at home and at work.
10. The serious health consequences of cigarette smoking, taking drugs, and drinking to excess are well known. The choice is yours.

The family The family, as a unit, is very important in relation to health. Social and personal behaviour is learned within the family. It is a powerful focus for learning about the health. Opportunities can be made available within the family setting to discuss difficult issues, or at least to listen to the problems.

The professionals Professional staff need to see their function as being about health as importantly as illness. They have an essential educational and leadership role with patients and the public. They can act as leaders to stimulate and facilitate change. From the point of view of health care they need to keep up to date and to continually improve their standards of care. Their curiosity and creativity should constantly be seeking ways to improve the public's health.

The community There are a wide range of issues which are the responsibility of the community. Community development projects are amongst the most powerful in improving health for the population group involved. They need to be able to ask a series of questions to ensure that health gets onto the agenda. Action plans need to be developed which involve the community as a whole, so that people know what to do, for example, 'on Monday morning'. Such plans require the need to communicate effectively, have a strategy in place, have trained staff available, and provide leadership.

The community, as patients and carers, brings considerable experience of both problems and solutions. We need to be able to listen and learn. The community, in the form of towns, cities, villages, offices, businesses, and streets, is a major educational setting from which real progress can be made. Such healthy communities provide opportunities for change and for individuals to develop and grow personally. There are numerous examples which show how community development projects have led to positive changes and given hope and fulfilment to those who felt isolated or even alienated. Such projects may not only put life and soul back into the community, but may also affect individuals in the same way.

At the occupational level The workplace is an important setting for improving health. Good health is good business. There is a real challenge to organizations to improve health by recognizing its value and by assisting the workforce from the point of view of health and safety.

At the national level The importance of developing a national health strategy has already been emphasized. The encouragement of partnerships, community development projects, and the assessment of the impact on health of cross-governmental policies, are all part of this. The state has a vital role, with others, in improving health, and good examples would include the reduction of road traffic accidents and the improvement of air quality. The importance of general education in the process of improving health needs underlining, and indeed it may be the most important factor of all.

Leadership To achieve the potential will need much hard work and commitment. It will also require leadership from those who feel passionately about bridging the gap between the actual and the possible. Such leaders must include all concerned, not just health professionals. Community leaders, including those from the religious communities, have an equally important role. It can be done if leadership is combined with a strong educational base and the provision of opportunities for both personal and community development.

11. Some conclusions

The remainder of the book discusses the issues outlined in greater detail. There is great optimism that such improvements can occur, and should occur. Future generations will judge our response to health and health care issues, not by the number of committees set up but by the outcome of our work. Cardinal Newman once said 'growth is the only evidence of life'. If we are to improve health it will require evidence of personal and institutional growth, evidence of vitality. We need such energy to achieve the potential.

Further reading

Callaghan, D. (1995). *What kind of life: the limits of medical progress.*
Evans, R. J. (1987). *Death in Hamburg. Society and politics in the cholera years 1830–1910.* Penguin.

2

Equity, poverty, and health for all

'If put in sufficiently general terms, the essence of the good society can be easily stated. It is that every member, regardless of gender, race or ethnic origin, should have access to a rewarding life.'* J. K. Galbraith, *The good society

In the opening chapter of this book, one of the first principles set out was health for all. The concept and the philosophy behind it provides both an overarching theme, and a vision of what might be achieved if the potential for improving health is to be realized. It is about having a life with meaning—an important concept and one which is particularly relevant when the subject of poverty is discussed. Under this one heading can be brought together many of the issues which really matter in improving the health of the public. These include the emphasis on health, the importance of equity, the relevance of partnerships, and the central need to involve patients and the public in health.

The World Health Organization (WHO) was not the first to use the slogan 'health for all'. In *Picture Post*, a weekly British magazine, Julian Huxley in the edition of 4 January 1941 discussed the need for improved health after the Second World War. In a prophetic article entitled 'health for all' he called for 'a healthy diet for all, everyone to have a chance to reach known health standards, public health as a positive service, health put on a family basis, a real family and population policy, and child welfare centres started everywhere'. The National Health Service was set up in the United Kingdom in 1948 and embodied many of these principles.

The WHO initiative began in Alma-Ata in Kazakhstan, in 1978, and this is a name which 'is synonymous with one of the great movements in public health history' (from *Alma Ata to the year 2000* WHO, 1988). The declaration emphasized the importance of equity, economic and social development, and of participation by the people in the process of improving health. In particular it stressed the crucial role of primary care and urged its development everywhere. In addition it encouraged each country to formulate national policies and strategies for health. To those who were around at the time it was a period of great vision and aspirations. It energized groups around the world to think about health in a different way. The Regions of the WHO took up the challenge and in 1984 the European Region launched its 38 targets. Then, it was revolutionary and led to a great deal of rethinking of health policy. The Health of the Nation strategy in England is thus in direct line from Alma-Ata. However, as the twenty-first century approaches, the strategy needs refreshing and revitalizing. At the present time, the WHO is in the process of undertaking such a revision and the new strategy will be completed by 1998. Around the world new ideas are being considered which will take Health for All into the next millennium.

Several issues which relate to the concept of health for all need to be considered. The first is whether, as a statement, it is too passive, and does not reflect the real need to involve people in improving health. It is for this reason that 'health *by* all' might be more appropriate. If this is accepted then it becomes clear that the mechanisms by which health is improved can only be effective through partnerships between all the agencies involved. This includes government, employers, employees, communities, local authorities, educational leaders, the voluntary sector, as well as individuals and families. Each of these needs to be party to the wish to change. Health for all should, therefore, be seen as everyone's responsibility, and not just that of health ministries or health professionals. If it is not, then much will be lost and the huge range of skills and expertise in the community will not be part of the process. The second issue which is raised is the importance of defining health, and being clear about the purpose of health. The WHO definition of health as 'a state of complete physical, mental and social well-being and not merely the absence of disease or infirmity' has been criticized for being too idealistic. However it does emphasize the holistic nature of health and its positive aspects. The WHO constitution continues, 'The health of all peoples is fundamental to the attainment of peace and is dependent on the fullest cooperation between individuals and states'. Once again, the importance of partnerships is stressed.

The purpose of health is equally difficult to define. Health can be a means or an end, though it is suggested that it is one component—albeit an important one—of quality of life. The concept of quality of life can be even more difficult to define and understand. For the purposes of this chapter it is the recognition of the gap between an individual's hopes and aspirations and reality. It is also therefore about potential and how it can be achieved. Health for all could equally well be expressed as 'quality of life for all'—health being one part of those events, circumstances, and situations which describe our own particular state of well-being. Living longer is not the only goal of improving health; improving quality of life can be the central one[1].

1. The determinants of health

In Chapter 1 these were briefly considered and to do so is an important first step in understanding health and how it might be improved.

1. Genetic factors Research over the last 20 years has shown how knowledge of our genetic make-up can allow us to understand the ways in which the body works, and what happens when it goes wrong. It is a most exciting area of biology. Increasingly it has become possible to identify a gene, or more likely several genes, which determine whether or not a particular disease will occur. With this understanding there comes the hope that treatment or preventative strategies will become available to control the problem. Gene therapy—or just as likely, the developing of new ways of treating illness—become possible.

2. The environment This includes a range of factors in the external world which may have an impact on health—air, soil, water, food, chemicals, radiation, and infectious diseases. These factors are all of great potential importance—a relevance recognized for some time. They are tied up with the concept of how we use resources in the natural world and how, in the process of development, we use them wisely. This is the thinking behind sustainable development in Agenda 21, and it is increasingly relevant to health.

Communicable diseases are a major threat to health. In most countries in the world they are the leading killers. Even in the developed countries they constitute a major problem which has not gone away. HIV infection, malaria, tuberculosis, hepatitis, and many others, old and new, pose new threats and challenge our strategies to contain them. Vaccination is one of the most cost-effective health interventions, but it is not sufficient. We need to remain always vigilant and able to deal with new problems with solutions ranging from effective hygiene measures at one end, to tracking antibiotic resistant organisms at the other.

3. Lifestyle This covers the very wide range of issues encompassing how we live and behave. These factors are very relevant to improving health. Cigarette smoking, for example, is the single most important cause of death in this country. Other lifestyle issues include excess alcohol consumption, drug taking, unsafe sex, violence, and risk-taking behaviour. To change these requires a personal decision, associated with a recognition that to do so will also depend on the environment and culture in which the change is to take place. Most of the problems are addictive and thus prevention is the most powerful weapon against them.

4. Social and economic factors It is well recorded that factors that influence health, income, housing, employment, and social class are all relevant. Poverty, deprivation, and unemployment all act against good health; for almost all illnesses, such factors are related to poorer health. For poverty this is true in both relative and absolute terms. The control of such factors is not wholly in the hands of the individual, and thus the role of the state or the employer becomes very important.

Of particular interest is the role of education in the prediction of health. In all societies and groups the level of educational attainment is readily correlated with levels of health. In the drive to improve health, educational improvement is a prerequisite.

5. *Health services* The contribution of health care to improving health is considerable, in curing patients, reducing disability, and improving quality of life. The factors which influence the outcome of health care will be detailed later. However it would be fair to say that the major influences on reaching health for all are more likely to be related to environment, lifestyle, and social and economic factors. This is most important when thinking about health at a strategic and population level.

2. Equity, equality, and health for all

One of the central features of health for all is its emphasis on equity and equality. Yet in spite of increasing interest in variations in health and health care and the inequities and inequalities which can occur, equity remains a significant issue. Over the past few years a number of reports have highlighted these long-standing and well-recognized variations[2]. The accurate recording of information on health—begun using Bills of Mortality in the seventeenth and eighteenth centuries, and developed further in the early nineteenth century—made such differences apparent. Yet they still exist.

There are therefore a number of determinants for health including biological and genetic factors, lifestyle and behaviour, the environment (including communicable diseases), social and economic factors, and health services. In all of these, the concepts of equity and equality are important, and the variations in health and health care which exist may be related to any of them—either alone or, more frequently, in combination. The term 'variations' is essentially neutral and is used to describe factual information about health and health care. However, the words 'equity' and 'equality' are often used interchangeably despite important distinctions between them. Equity is about fairness and justice, and implies that everyone should have an opportunity to attain their full potential for health. Equality, on the other hand, is about comparisons between individuals and communities of the level of health or ability to obtain access to health care. Some inequalities may be unavoidable, and therefore generally not considered unfair, while others might be avoided and are thus considered inequitable.

Natural, biological, and genetic variations may have unavoidable (though very important) health inequalities related to them. Lifestyle and behaviour patterns chosen by individuals, for example, cigarette smoking can also result in inequalities in health. In some instances health promotion activities, if selectively taken up, may even increase the inequalities—but again this might not be considered inequitable as they are the result of personal choice. However, lifestyle and behaviour that is not freely chosen, and which results in poor health, might be considered as avoidable and thus inequitable. Health inequalities arising from the level of resources, housing conditions, dangerous working conditions, or exposure to environmental hazards, would be examples of these. Inadequate access to health care or other public services might also be inequitable if the cause was avoidable and the result was inequality: such factors might include transport, lack of information, or inaccessibility of information as a result of language difficulties. There are also inequalities in the range of facilities available, and considerable variations in quality of care and outcomes of treatment across the country.

In considering the actions which might be required to ensure that inequities were reduced, a group was set up in

England in 1995 to review the evidence of the effectiveness of interventions within key health areas of the nation (coronary heart disease and stroke, accidents, mental health, cancers, and HIV and sexual health)[3]. One of the main conclusions of this report was that there was little published literature on the subject, and what there was gave few pointers to effective action. Thus while the issue is of considerable importance, and the National Health Service in the United Kingdom is strongly committed to tackling inequities, much more research is required. In the meantime targeting of resources to meet particular needs, together with action at a social and economic level and information provision, offer some ways forward.

Distributive justice

So far so good. Defining equity and equality is relatively easy. The difficulty comes in two respects:

1. How do you decide what is fair or just? Are there any principles which can be used?
2. How can this be put into practice?

These questions are general ones and relate not only to equity but to priority setting, rationing, and the way resources are used. The central principle is the value base from which decisions are made. It is this which determines what is fair or just. Decisions are made even more difficult because of the uncertainty of outcome. Some other issues are relevant:

1. Most problems are complex, and there is no right answer.
2. Choices need to be made within fixed resources.
3. The knowledge base is only one component of decision making.
4. Logical argument is only one part of the process.
5. The public view needs to be considered.
6. There is always room for differences of opinion.

Some ideas on fairness, justice, and equity Such issues have been discussed since the time of Plato and there are no commonly agreed views as to the basis of decision making. Jurisprudence—the study of the philosophical and ethical foundation of the law—provides a range of theories (for example, Hart's 'Concept of law'[4], Rawls' 'Theory of justice'[5]). There is a general agreement that:

1. Each person should have an equal right to basic liberties, for example, freedom of speech, assembly, thought.
2. Each person has a right to equal opportunities, especially through education. However, thereafter there is less consensus. Most of the health issues related to equity come under the category of 'distributive justice'—that is, how benefits, resources, and burdens of society are distributed to each individual. The rules define how society co-operates and these relate directly to the values in society. Such resources may be distributed:
   (a) to each person an equal share;
   (b) to each person according to individual needs;
   (c) to each person according to individual efforts;
   (d) to each person according to societal contributions;
   (e) to each person according to merit.

Very different choices would be made depending on the option selected. Such principles are mutually incompatible. They are however closely related to some basic ethical principles, namely:

(a) autonomy—rights of the individual;
(b) beneficence—doing good;
(c) non-malevolence—not doing harm;
(d) utility—the greatest good, the greatest number;
(e) equity—justice and fairness.

These too, in some circumstances, are mutually incompatible and conflicting.

Putting equity into practice

How can such principles be put into practice, and is it possible to define an operating framework? In reviewing such issues from a national or public health perspective, consider how similar issues are dealt with by the practising doctor. The problem faced by the doctor in the clinical situation of deciding, with the full involvement of the patient, the appropriate choice of treatment, and how best to use resources, is analogous to that faced by the public health professional or the politician, who has to deal with problems of a different order. The following questions are asked by the patient and, by analogy, the public:

1. **What is the problem?**
   The diagnosis.
2. **What does it mean?**
   The prognosis.
3. **What might be done?**
   The range and choice of interventions and treatments available.
4. **What should be done?**
   Decision on the appropriate action based on the possible benefits
5. **How will you know if it is worthwhile?**
   The measurement of the outcome.
6. **Will you keep things under review?**
   Redefining the problem.

Using this clinical model, the implications for public health and policy making become apparent and follow the same stages:

1. The definition of the problem (diagnosis) and a marshalling of the evidence is the first step. A critical and knowledge-based review of those health problems which are of particular concern is carried out.
2. Based on this, identification of the health needs of the population is established. Participation of the public is required at this stage in defining priorities.
3. Review of all possible choices for intervention (prevention, treatment, rehabilitation, and so on) with possible benefits, disadvantages, and costs.
4. Appropriate choices then need to be made on the basis of this information. These will take into account the

uncertainties, with the evidence and the fact that judgement will be required. This is the key stage and, just as in the clinical model, this is when public involvement is essential. Having made the decision resources are allocated and treatment is begun.
5. The outcome is defined and the intervention is regularly assessed. The important evaluation stage is built in from the beginning.
6. The problems are redefined at regular intervals.

This model at least provides a framework with which to test the mechanism by which equity is put in practice. It emphasizes the importance of education and of providing opportunities for action and involvement. All models are simplifications of complex situations, and all have inherent problems. This particular model, based on the analogy with clinical practice, stresses the need to define the problem and to involve the public in choices. In the end however judgement will always be required to make the final decision. This is perhaps why 'Justice' is usually depicted blindfold, holding a balance, and weighing up the evidence in as objective a way as possible.

Conclusions on equity

Equity is about fairness and justice and is at the heart of health for all. It should be distinguished from the related concept of equality. There are several different principles of distributive justice and the choice made depends on the values selected. Such principles may be incompatible and conflicting. Variations in health and health care exist. To tackle this effectively requires further research. A most important issue however is reaching a consensus of the values to be used.

3. Poverty and health

Of all the determinants of health, why should poverty be picked out for particular attention? What makes poverty special in relation to health? The impetus for these questions lies in the fact that poverty, worldwide, is frequently associated with poor health. Although it is not readily definable it is one of a number of determinants of health, and has a profound effect on well-being. The concept of poverty is often mixed up with other terms such as deprivation, inequality, disadvantage, alienation, and marginalization. These are important social and economic factors, which together with the other determinants of health contribute to overall well-being. Poverty must therefore be seen in this context, as one factor in determining health.

Poverty and health have been seen as related for many years. As Adam Smith pointed out in *The Wealth of Nations*:

> But poverty, though it does not prevent the generation, is extremely unfavourable to the rearing of children . . . It is not uncommon I have been frequently told, in the Highlands of Scotland for a mother who has borne 20 children not to have 2 alive . . . This great mortality, however, will everywhere be found chiefly among the children of the common people, who cannot afford to tend them with the same care as those of a better station.

Defining poverty

One key problem is to arrive at a clear definition of poverty, and to consider what action might be taken to alleviate it. The following definition, set out in a series of statements brings together much of the writing on the subject, and in that sense is not original:

> Poverty is a term which describes the state of an individual or a group, where there is a lack of resources which significantly affects health and well-being. The lack of resources may include money, material possessions, emotional and psychological support, environmental protection, education, opportunities, shelter, housing, information, and so on.
>
> Poverty can be absolute or relative. Absolute poverty (Rowntree called this primary poverty[8]) exists where the lack of resources may result in an inability to provide adequate food, shelter, and essentials of life, which may result in a life-threatening state. Relative poverty is measured by comparing individuals or groups, and relating them to some norm, defined locally, nation-

ally, or internationally. Whichever way it is defined, it identifies a gap between what is and what might be, and thus the potential for improvement.

Poverty for any individual is not necessarily a static state and can change with age, employment status, disability, and other factors. It is thus a potentially reversible situation.

Poverty may have several consequences and a variety of interrelated terms are used for this purpose. They include deprivation, alienation, inequalities, social exclusion, disadvantage, and marginalization. These alone, or in combination, can lead to loss of well-being, a poorer quality of life, and a life without meaning.

Poverty is associated with other related concepts such as social class, culture, education, employment, and the nature of the environment. Each of these can compound the problem.

The income time line

It is possible to consider the well-being of an individual (or perhaps even a community) as a moveable point which draws a line over the lifespan of the person. The position is likely to vary over time and be dependent on age, social circumstances, income, educational opportunities, employment status, illness, disability, and so on.

Substantial shifts may occur up or down, and relate to major life events—for example, relative, marital breakdown, change in employment status, birth of a child, episode of illness (Figs 2.1 and 2.2). Statistics on poverty bear out the

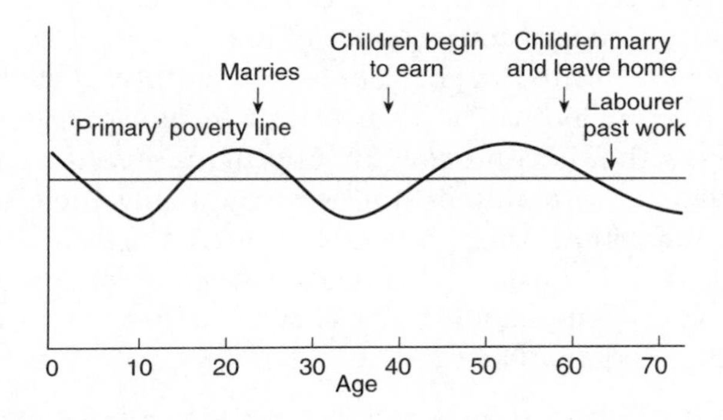

Fig. 2.1—The line of poverty[8]

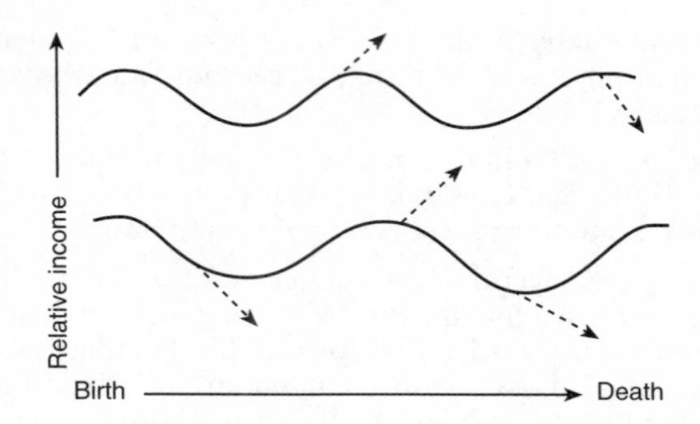

Fig. 2.2—The income time line for two different people: position on the line reflects current income. The higher the point, the better the quality of life. Arrows show that significant income changes may occur.

fact that there is significant income mobility: poverty is reversible, and not inevitable. The mechanisms to effect the change relate to the causes: social structure, employment and educational opportunities, level of health, and so on. It is likely that multiple mechanisms will be required to deal with the problem. One consequence of this is that individuals must take an active part in helping to create the opportunities, and be willing to take them. Individuals or groups may move up or down, but relative differences in income and social status may remain. What is key is that everyone has the opportunity to achieve their full potential and have the highest possible level of health and quality of life.

A further general issue which is often raised is whether or not poverty, and as a consequence of it, ill health, is related to the individual, or to the environment or culture in which the person lives, or both. The answer to this question will give clues as to the mechanisms for improving health. Though more evidence is required, studies suggest that the environment is important, though personal factors are clearly also relevant. A. J. Toynbee, in his book *A study of history*, makes an important point about the 'proletariat' which can be translated into alienation:

For [proletarianism] is a state of feeling rather than a matter of outward circumstance . . . we defined it for our purpose, as a social element or group which in some way is 'in' but not 'of' any given society at any given stage in that societies history . . . The true hallmark of the [proletarian] is neither poverty nor humble birth but a consciousness—and a resentment which this consciousness inspires—of being disinherited from his ancestral place in society and being unwanted in a community which is his rightful home; and this subjective [proletarianism] is not incompatible with the possession of material assets.

This quotation sets out clearly the feelings and consequences of alienation.

Some questions

The description of the relationships between poverty and health take us only so far. Some questions remain:

1. What is the mechanism by which poverty or deprivation can cause illness and disease? Are there molecular mechanisms which can explain the effects? It is possible to suggest some hypotheses which could be tested.
2. What are the ethical issues which surround poverty and deprivation in a developed country? How does society resolve its own conscience in this matter? What are the values which are most important?
3. What further research needs to be carried out? Do we know enough from an epidemiological point of view, but less about effective methods for the implementation of policies?

Tackling poverty

If the objective is to narrow the gap between what is and what might be, and improve the quality of life and the sense of well-being, how can this be done? As poverty is in most instances a relative concept it is unlikely that the gap will be eliminated, and as Galbraith argues, there may even be a need to have such differences in society[7]. It should be obvious that there are no simple solutions to the problem. As has been described, the income of individuals may vary from time to time. For this reason different interventions may be required at different times, for example, in childhood and old age. It is complex and many different agencies and groups are involved. To effect change it is necessary to consider material issues, psychological implications, and environmental and cultural factors. To tackle these will require a range of initiatives (there is not likely to be a single solution), and it is necessary to consider both the individual and the community. Community development projects, where people are involved in improving the local environment, can provide a very useful vehicle within which a wide variety of approaches can be used. These might include:

- targeting resources and expertise appropriately
- developing educational opportunities—perhaps the most important
- appropriate tax and benefit measures
- changing the environment
- providing adequate housing.

These measures are essentially external, providing both a better environment and opportunities for all. They all attempt to improve the quality of life and self esteem.

However there is another side of the coin, and that is the ability of an individual or a community to profit from these opportunities. If the 'soul' is to be put back into the community, and individuals regain a sense of worth, then they too have a responsibility. Initiatives such as Our Healthier Nation provide the vehicle for both personal and community development. It is neither a National Health Service or a Government initiative—it is for all to be involved.

4. Conclusions

To achieve change and improve health is both a science and an art. Suffice it to say that several different approaches will need to be used if success is to be achieved. Our understanding of health and illness, and their determinants, is central to this. Health for all is not just a slogan. It is a way of thinking about improving health for the population as a whole. Those who are at particular disadvantage require specific care and consideration. Poverty, no matter how it is defined, is a particular issue which needs special attention. The quest for health is the quest for social justice.

References

1. Calman, K. C. (1984). Quality of life in cancer patients—an hypothesis. *J Med Ethics*, **10**, 124–7.
2. (1992). *Inequalities and health. The Black Report and the health divide.* Penguin Books.
3. Department of Health. (1995). *Variations in health. What can the Department of Health and the NHS do?*
4. Hart, H. L. A. (1961). *The concept of law.* Oxford University Press.
5. Rawls, J. (1972). *A theory of justice.* Oxford University Press.
6. Downie, R. S. and Calman, K. C. (1994). *Healthy respect*, 2nd edn. Oxford University Press.
7. Galbraith, J. K. (1996). *The good society. The human agenda.* Sinclair-Stevenson, London.
8. Rowntree, S. (1902). *Poverty. A study of town life.*

3

The health of the nation

In the introductory chapter of this book, one of the principles outlined was the need to have a national strategy to improve health. Between 1991 and 1997 the 'Health of the Nation' fulfilled that function. It has now been developed further and broadened into 'Our Healthier Nation'. Following a discussion on the principles behind the first of these initiatives, the second stage will be outlined.

1. Key areas and targets

The Health of the Nation strategy represents a major policy statement, the objective of which is to improve health in England. It follows in the footsteps of the 'Health for All' initiative, but takes it further, presenting a number of new dimensions. It was first published in 1992, and over the past five years there has been considerable effort and activity in moving towards the targets. While it is far too early to comment on the long-term achievement of these targets, the early indications are encouraging. The objective, as always, is to improve health, health care, and quality of life, and to ensure that it is not simply adding years to life, but life to years. Its objective is clearly based on improving the public's health.

One of the important features of the Health of the Nation strategy is that it restricts itself to a limited number of key areas and targets. It began with five key areas; coronary heart disease and stroke; cancers; accidents; mental illness;

AIDS, HIV, and sexual health. Such a limited number, with the accompanying total of 27 health targets, simplify the process of managing the implementation. By setting targets it has been possible to give direction to the process, to facilitate discussion of the magnitude of the change required, to ensure that appropriate resources are available, and to allow monitoring of the process. Such targets have been invaluable in looking at the progress of the strategy. Each of the targets have been reviewed on a very regular basis, and consideration given as to whether they should be modified or changed. The philosophy throughout has been to engage the wider community through partnerships and joint working. Without this the Health of the Nation will not achieve its objectives.

One of the key features of the whole process was the setting up of a Cabinet Sub-Committee, chaired by a senior politician, to co-ordinate the effort and to oversee the process. This has unquestionably been the signal that the political will was there to improve health. The Committee has met on a regular basis over the last few years, and has considered all the key areas. It has allowed interdepartmental discussions, thus making clear that the Health of the Nation is a truly interdepartmental issue. But it goes beyond that. The Health of the Nation is not about the National Health Service or the Government or any individual organization. One of the successes of the Health of the Nation is that it has brought together a very wide range of groups—organizations both voluntary and governmental—to ensure that the health of the public is improved. Once again, it emphasizes the importance of health by all, rather than health for all.

In the initial period following publication of the Report, a variety of practice manuals on each of the key areas was published, covering a very broad range of interests. These have been supplemented over the years by publications on particular areas of the Health of the Nation, and on the ways in which it can be monitored and improved. These have included the publication of a Public Health Common Data Set, a geographically based information service, on progress towards the targets, and a very wide range of documentation for all the interest groups involved. This has ensured regular information to the public and to the professionals involved. A regular newsletter entitled *Target* is also produced. One of the most important of the Reports published was 'Variations in health' which looked at the five key areas of the Health of the Nation and the extent to which variations occurred within the National Health Service, and the ways in which such variations and inequalities could be reduced. The conclusion was that while such variations were known to exist, the published literature on effective interventions was sparse.

2. Delivering the strategy

The Health of the Nation has been delivered using three related approaches. Fundamental to all has been the development of the concept of:

- healthy settings
- healthy alliances or partnerships
- healthy groups.

From the point of view of healthy settings this has included a considerable amount of activity in establishing the idea of healthy cities, workplaces, schools, homes, hospitals, environments, communities, villages, and prisons. This has undoubtedly captured the imagination of a variety of groups and a great deal of activity has gone on at local level in schools, workplaces, and in communities. Unquestionably one of the most exciting areas is being able to see these community development projects go forward, and to experience the great enthusiasm of individuals within a community who really do wish to change health. The role of primary care within this has of course been important, and the primary care team and general practitioners have done a great deal locally to ensure that such developments do progress. The general practitioners surgery is an important focus of such activity. Religious leaders also have an essential part to play. Within the community they are highly respected, and can bring the community together. They generally have access to premises, and are able to influence in a positive way the particular group involved.

One of the more interesting developments from the Health Service point of view has been the concept of a 'healthy hospital'. A number of acute hospitals have taken this forward with initiatives, not just for the patients and for their future rehabilitation in the community, but also for the staff, and the provision for them of appropriate facilities in terms of food, exercise and staff welfare. The National Health Service is the biggest workforce in Europe, and by using the Health of the Nation as a trigger for improving the health of its workers, there is then enormous scope for improving health generally. With this in mind specific teaching packs have been developed for hospital doctors.

Another important development has been the use of healthy alliances or partnerships. Partnerships within towns and cities, the education departments, environment, business and commerce, and the voluntary organizations have all shown how by working together health and the environment can be considerably improved. Publications on healthy alliances have been produced and a wide range of communities have advanced this concept. Minority groups within the communities have been included, and the use of local representatives to help these people understand the key health problems in the community and how best to deal with them, has been important. So, vital steps to improving the health of a number of ethnic minority groups have been taken. While much of this has been going on within towns, and in particular within inner cities, it should not be forgotten that rural areas are just as important. Rural deprivation and problems of communication are very real. For this reason a number of projects have concentrated on this aspect.

The third concept to be considered is that of healthy groups. The most obvious one, and the one in which most work has been done is the Health of the Young Nation. The health of adolescents, in particular, presents great challenges, and there has been much activity in this area. The health of young people is of special concern and it is in this group that major behavioural patterns are established. This has involved considerable work through a variety of healthy alliances and, in particular, co-operation with Departments of Education. As part of triggering the effort in this area a series of awards, Health Alliance Awards, have been instigated. They have shown how across the country groups of all types have been working together to improve the health of the nation. Specific interest has focused on those who are disabled, and this has provided some especially interesting areas of community development

There has been considerable attention over the years to the health of women, and programmes are well established in this area. There has been less work however on men's health, though over the last few years this has attained greater attention. Men do have particular health problems and seem much more reluctant than women to use the resources available.

A final area for mention is that of work in the workplace—an important aspect which has once again involved a wide variety of groups looking at the health of their workforce and ensuring that this is taken into account in developing new initiatives.

Much of the information produced has been in written form, but experiments with other methods have taken place. These have included video and audio material, discussion groups, and, of course, electronically through the Internet. This latter is one way in which young men, who seem to have particular difficulty getting access to health information, may be encouraged to come forward and take action.

3. The results so far

On a regular basis the progress has been evaluated, and the results published and reviewed widely. In general, advances have been made towards achieving the targets, many of which do not have a target date until the next century. For example, there have been substantial reductions in coronary heart disease, mortality, and breast cancer, and lung cancer in men (see Figs 3.1–3.3). However, there are a number of areas which continue to cause concern including the rise in suicides (particularly in young men), problems with cigarette smoking in adolescents, excessive alcohol consumption, increasing obesity, and a lack of physical activity. These are all very important lifestyle areas which clearly require greater effort. As far as physical activity is concerned, for example, as a nation we now take less exercise than we did some years ago, but there have been a number of fascinating initiatives, again at local level, that constitute an advance. These have included alliances between general practitioners and local leisure centres to ensure that exercise is prescribed for

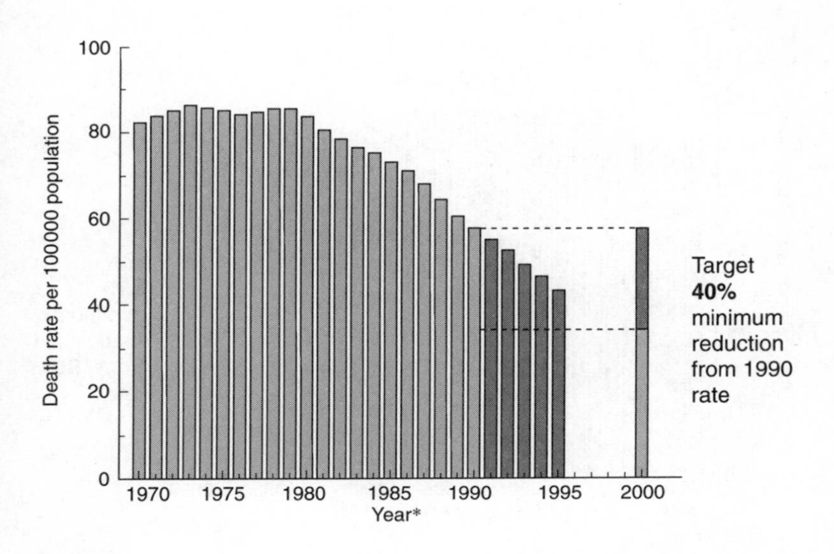

Fig. 3.1—Death rates‡ for coronary heart disease in all persons aged under 65 in England, 1969–96; and the target for the year 2000.

those who need it. Promoting walking, both in towns and the countryside has been an interesting part of this. These experiments of encouraging people to think more about themselves, and particularly about their body weight, with a combination of diet and exercise, are beginning to bear fruit. The challenge however remains, and it is an important challenge. Over the last four years it has become clear that things can change for the better, and that once the public recognizes the importance of change, and that health is something to be valued, then it is remarkable to see how things progress.

The Health of the Nation has been in place for five years, and it must always be remembered that it is in a one-stage, long-term strategy. But the early results are sufficiently encouraging to say that health and well-being can be improved by bringing together a wide range of people,

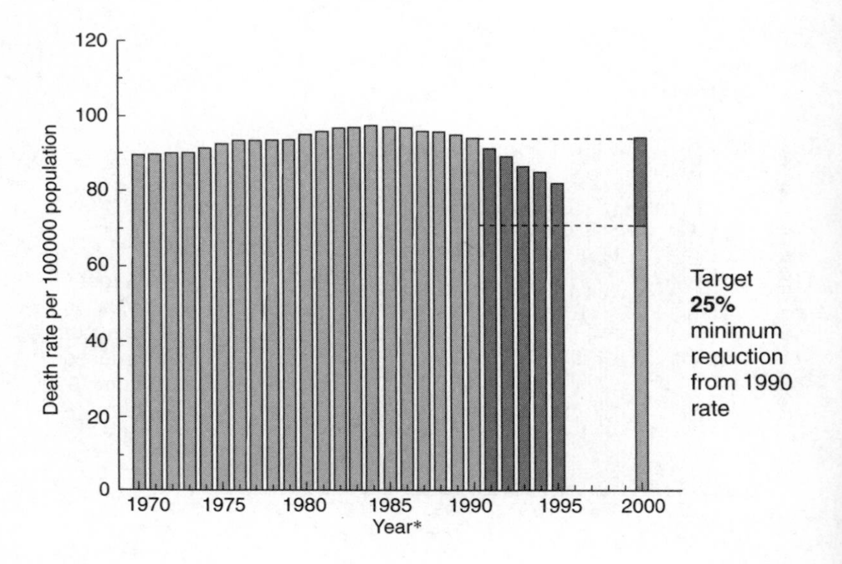

Fig. 3.2—Death rates‡ for cancer of the breast in women aged 50–69 in England, 1969–96; and the target for the year 2000.

and by using the skills and expertise of the population as a whole.

4. Our healthier nation

The Health of the Nation strategy is currently being re-examined and advanced under the new title of 'Our Healthier Nation'. This new strategy, while retaining some of the the existing targets will set a new direction, emphasizing social exclusion, inequalities in health, and the importance of housing, employment, and the environment in improving health and well-being. New targets will also be developed, with greater emphasis on local priorities and particular stress on the health of children (especially healthy schools), health in the workplace, and health within the elderly population. It will be an 'across-

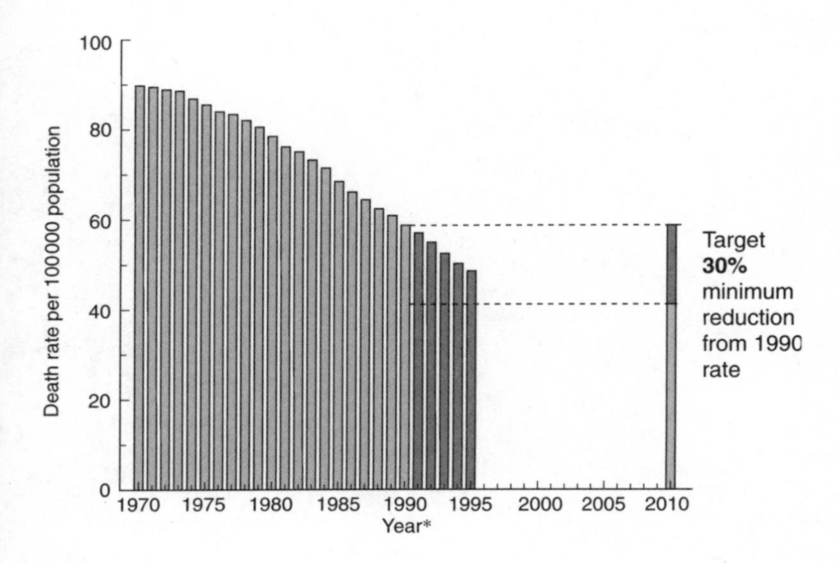

Fig. 3.3—Death rates‡ for lung cancer in males aged under 75 in England, 1969–96; and the target for the year 2000.

government' strategy focused on improving the outcomes of interventions to change the health of the population. Some of this will be taken forward at community level through 'healthy living centres' which will emphasize lifestyle changes. Some will be developed through 'health action zones', bringing together a range of partners to improve health, health care, and the delivery of services.

4

Public and patient involvement in health and health care

***'I know of no safe depository of the ultimate powers of society but the people themselves; and if we think them not enlightened enough to exercise their control with a wholesome discretion, the remedy is not to take it from them, but to inform their discretion.'* Thomas Jefferson (letter to W. C. Jarvis, 28 September 1820)**

1. Introduction

It has been argued at the start of this book that it is impossible to change health or health care without the involvement of the public. Indeed it is both a truism, and a central principle. It is about realizing the potential for health—the theme of this book. Personal involvement in health care is also important, not only for the patient or the carer, but for the taxpayer and consumer, to ensure value for money. This chapter will therefore consider several broad issues:

- How do the public perceive health?
- What are patient expectations of health and health care?
- How can we ensure patient choice and involvement in health care?
- How can we ensure public involvement in the allocation of resources and choices of health care?
- What is the role of the public in health issues?
- How can we best communicate risks to the public?

- What is the role of the media in health and health care?
- What is the role of the public in professional education?

A variety of different words can be used to describe the kind or degree of involvement envisaged: they include empowerment, participation, and ownership. Each has a different slant but they all have relevance to the topic, and will be used in different places in this chapter. They all add up to the fact that issues of health and health care belong to people, assisted by professionals, and not the other way round.

It could be argued that, together with the chapter on equity, these are the most important chapters in this book. If the public are not, or cannot be fully involved in decisions about their own health then an opportunity has been lost. The theme of this book is that there is an unfulfilled potential, the power of which can be released if individuals, communities, and populations recognize the importance of health and begin to take action. This chapter will outline some of the difficulties and constraints against achieving this, and will suggest some ways in which involvement can be improved. But first a discussion on some general themes which are relevant throughout the chapter is required.

One way of illustrating the importance of the topic is to describe the apocryphal 'add an egg' advertising story. When cake mixes were first introduced the housewife only had to add water and mix. This did not feel right and there was no satisfaction in the finished product, no ownership. For this reason the manufacturers reformulated the product so that an egg had to be added. This increased involvement and ensured increasing sales of the product.

2. Some general issues

Who are the public?

This is a central problem. Whenever the question of representation arises, whenever there is a need for members of the public or patients, who is to be chosen? Professionals, of course, are also citizens and thus members of the public, and therefore potential or actual patients. They have a right to be involved and their personal input cannot be dismissed, though clearly it is not sufficient. But take as an example a general practice somewhere in England. The practice team have decided that it would be a positive move to set up a patient participation group, and they advertise this locally. Some 20 people turn up to the first meeting out of a practice population of 12 500. How representative are they, and how much notice should be placed on their views? Another example would be that of a major committee on developing guidelines for patient care wishing to involve patients. How should it be done? Who would represent patients? These are just two examples of a very general problem. As a member of the public, who would I like to represent me and in whom would I have confidence? Single-issue groups or pressure groups bring very special expertise to discussions, but they might not be able to see the broader picture. At the national level the democratic process sees to it that our political representatives fulfil this function. In recent years the role of citizen juries, patient panels, and broadly selected groups have provided routes into this important area. The role of community health councils is an important part of this.

There are however no easy answers to the questions posed and each one may have a different solution. What we need to do is share good practice and learn from each other. Most importantly we should start now to begin the process.

The special role of women

Throughout this book the special role of women in health is emphasized. In relation to involvement in health their role is crucial. As consumers of health care it is generally women who look after the family, take children to the health service, and, as the principal carers, make most use of social care. They make decisions within the family about lifestyle, food, and health, and it is this role which makes their perception of health and assessment of risks so important.

Why should we involve the public and patients?

So far the assumption has been made that it is worthwhile ensuring that the public have a role. But why? First, the public need to have ownership of their own health and that of their community if we are to see significant change. Otherwise any initiative will be seen as 'top down' rather than 'bottom up'. The public are highly sophisticated (they must be as I am one of them), they have enormous experience of life and of illness, and as citizens have a right to be involved. We need the power and the experience of the public if we are to change health and take the right decisions about resource allocation and the provision and range of services. It is true that the public need information from professionals upon which to base decisions and make informed choices. That is a necessary, but not sole part of the process. It is essential that patients are involved and participate fully in decisions about their health and health care. They need to be given options and to take part in choices about treatment and rehabilitation. Professionals need to recognize the great value of this process and the relevance of patient experience.

How do we involve them?

Much depends on the issue and whether or not we need an 'experienced' person or a 'generic' one. For example, if one is looking for a public representative for an AIDs committee, is it necessary to have someone who is HIV positive? Or for a group dealing with the problems of the elderly, is it helpful to have someone over the age of 70? And what does involvement really mean? Attendance at a few committee meetings or a real part in decision making? As always there may be no right answer, but the questions need to be asked.

These comments represent a few of the general issues which are often raised when this subject is discussed. The next few sections deal with more specific issues.

3. Perceptions of health

One of the most important issues in determining health is how we perceive health and illness. The objectives of this section are firstly to analyze perceptions, secondly to examine how we learn about health, and thirdly to consider how we can change perceptions of health and improve both quality of life and health of the population. The importance of the subject cannot be underestimated: a brief consideration of smoking, HIV infection, food safety, nutrition, and accidents all show clearly how changing perceptions of an individual, or of a group of individuals, will modify the way we think about health and thus affect the action that we might take to alter behaviour. Our perception is related to what we know and how that knowledge is translated into behaviour. Many of the current health problems which we face, such as coronary heart disease, stroke, cancers, and accidents, are all related to lifestyle. Thus, perceptions of health may be one of the most important barriers to its improvement. How patients and the public perceive health is a first step in ensuring their involvement in decision making. To take some specific examples:

1. Cigarette smoking is well known to be harmful to the health of both the individual and of those breathing in the smoke. Yet we know that the incidence of smoking in teenage girls remains stable or rising, and that their perception is that smoking is not harmful and indeed a positive thing to do.
2. A second issue would be HIV infection and the importance of safe sex. There are a very large number of myths surrounding HIV infection, many of which determine our perception of risk, and this may or may nor result in changing behaviour.

3. In terms of food—whether in relation to safety, hygiene, or nutritional value—the public, and many professionals, are unable to separate myth from reality, and their perceptions of risks once again determine behaviour.
4. From crossing the road to using seat belts, accidents, as a final example, show clearly how both children and adults take specific care about reducing injury, by altering their behaviour. Thus the perception of the risk is obviously important.

In this next section three issues will be considered: the subject of knowledge will first be discussed; followed by a review of perception and the need to understand change; and finally an analysis of tools available to assist the change.

The knowledge base

The first issue to consider is that of knowledge. Knowledge itself is, of course, inert. It is the perception of that knowledge which is subsequently translated into behaviour. The knowledge base from which the individual draws perceptions is therefore crucial and may itself be inadequate in that the information required is not always available. There may be ignorance of the knowledge, or the knowledge itself may be false. In addition, knowledge given by different parties or organizations may be conflicting. Thus if our perceptions of health and healthy lifestyles are based on the knowledge which we have, then there are a number of reasons why that knowledge base may be insufficient to meet our needs. For this reason it is not surprising that people's perceptions of health may vary considerably. The importance of stories, anecdotes, and 'old wives' tales are part of this.

The development of perception

Secondly, perception may be said to be the interpretation of reality by an individual group or community. It is how we perceive reality that matters. The way in which a group of individuals watching the same television programme can react in varying ways shows clearly how differently individuals can interpret what they see. When Emmanuel Kant said 'we see things not as they are, but as we are', he showed enormous insight into the problem of perception. We all see things differently, sometimes pessimistically and sometimes optimistically, but the variations between us are enormous. Part of perception of course is common sense, and the original meaning of common sense was the integration of the five senses into a common experience, that process being affected by previous experience.

The perception of health varies considerably, for example, between children and adults, and between men and women. Different subgroups of the population such as ethnic minorities also perceive health and health issues, such as access to health care, quite differently. There is a special role for women who, in general, are the carers and the source of information and wisdom during emergencies, and who retain the folk memory of how to deal with health issues. Messages about health are readily passed between generations in this way.

An alternative way of looking at this is to see how we perceive risk. A number of situations which are readily seen in almost any newspaper or television programme concern the public's views about risk. Whether this relates to HIV infection, food, or an environmental hazard, the assessment of risk is of course not easy. The Royal Society have recently published a book entitled *Risk analysis, perception and management*. The British Medical Association's book *Living with risk* summarizes many of the issues. Issues of risk are of course viewed differently between groups of patients, the public, professionals, and politicians. These differences may well relate to conflicts at the time of making decisions. A more recently recognized piece of work raises perhaps the more important issue from the pubic's point of view—risk communication. This will be discussed in a subsequent section.

Perception therefore relates to the background experience and the perspective which each individual brings to it. In changing our perceptions there is often a personal cost related to that change and there is the added complication of the time factor. For example, the risk in relation to cigarette smoking may seem to be so far away that the perception is that there is no need to change. Short-term and long-term implications of perceptions need to be taken into account.

The growth of knowledge and tools for change

This leads to a discussion about how we learn about health. We learn in a remarkable variety of ways—through books, the family, media, the educational system, and from friends and role models. Of these, friends and role models are considered to be among the most powerful. Footballers, pop stars, and models act as role models and can change the behaviour and attitudes of large numbers of the population. Each person's value base is important as a determinant of health. It is values which alter perception, and these are related to basic human values, society's values, our own personal values, and, where appropriate, professional values. Values in society vary enormously in cultural terms, for example, in relation to women or homosexuals, and in political terms, in relation to the social or health care system which is in operation. Our own personal values relate to upbringing, education, peer pressure, and personal experiences related to religion, culture, and any special knowledge which we may have, for example, by being a doctor or a teacher.

In trying to change health perhaps the most important thing about learning is what the learner already knows. This means that we have to begin changing health from the point where the individual actually *is*. If we try to change health based on what *we* think people should know then we will be missing perhaps the most important aspect of learning. This section emphasizes therefore the importance of role models, peer groups, and an understanding of an individual's or a group's perception of a particular health issue or lifestyle pattern.

To change the perception of health, and thus behaviour, is not easy. It may require the individual to change personally, but it may also necessitate social and political change. The individual or the group have to participate in change and see health in a positive way as something which fulfils their own potential, and not as a negative, punitive issue. They must feel involved—and ownership is central to this. They must feel that it is valuable to change. What we require therefore is an educational strategy which is acceptable to the population, understandable, and contains consistent messages. It should be based on previous experience and grounded in the knowledge base and values of that individual or group. Imposed values are unlikely to change behaviour. Related to this is the importance of the consistency of the message. A recent British social attitudes survey noted that 71 per cent of experts disagreed about food advice and that 42 per cent of the population ignored food advice. This indicates the magnitude of the task ahead. What is required therefore is to try to get things into perspective and to develop tools for change based on appropriate models, for example, an educational model, a social-change model, or a problem-based model. This last model, if associated with a knowledge of the current position of that individual or group in their perception of the issues, may be the most useful.

Change, however, comes at a cost, which may be of a personal nature related to resources or to time. From the point of view of time and change there is a need to consider age and perspective, and this has both short-term and long-term implications. There may be an appropriate time to change and it may be difficult to identify what the right time is. It is known, for example, that a consultation between a doctor and a patient is a very powerful time to discuss issues of changing behaviour.

Implicit within this is the importance of research and development. It is the knowledge base which will change perception. If that knowledge base is inadequate then we must ensure that the appropriate research is carried out to strengthen the knowledge base. The media have an important role to play in this, which will be discussed later.

It is possible therefore to conclude, at this stage, that:

1. Perceptions of health are important in changing health.
2. We need to understand how people learn about health.
3. Effective models and tools for change are required.
4. Role models, the media, and the knowledge base are central to changes in health.

The way we perceive health and how that is translated into behaviour is thus one of the most important issues facing public health at the present time. It is essential that our knowledge base is extended and that an active programme of research is undertaken in this important area.

4. Expectations of health and health care

One hundred years ago expectations of health and health care were small. When illness occurred there was an inevitability about the expectations of both life and death, with little available to influence the outcome. The doctor gave advice and perhaps treatment, much of which was ineffective. Now, with the enormous developments in medical and scientific research, many diseases are treatable, if not curable; diagnostic processes are clearer; and the public may expect that if they are ill, then treatment will be available which will result in rapid cure. Similarly, when matters of health are raised, for example, with immunization or environmental factors which impact on health, expectations are that the process of change is simple, that there will be no side-effects or long-term consequences, and that a magic wand is available which makes new developments problem free. But is this reasonable? It is certainly true that effective treatment is available for many conditions but a number of factors need to be recognized:

1. Even something relatively simple, such as the use of an antibiotic for an infected throat, may not be effective in all cases (a second antibiotic may be required) and there may be side-effects. Hence the importance for the patient of information and choice.
2. Sometimes the diagnosis is difficult to make. Putting a label on a set of symptoms may not solve the problem. This is particularly the case when symptoms are non-specific and the tests inconclusive. It may not be possible to have a clear diagnosis in all cases. The interpretation of X-rays, electrocardiographs, and laboratory tests all carry a margin of error.
3. It is for this reason, a quite understandable one, that opinions of doctors may vary. Judgements can differ and doctors are not infallible, which is why systems of audit, clinical review, and case conferences are so important to ensure that no particular factor has been missed or overlooked. It is also why communication with the patient about possible uncertainty is vital in ensuring that expectations are not unreasonable.
4. Illness still occurs in spite of advances in medical technology: infection remains a problem, cancer has not been eliminated, heart disease is still a major killer. There is sometimes a wish that such illnesses could be banished or cures be available in all cases. While there have been enormous improvements in care, medical science has not yet solved all the problems. Relapses will occur even in the best treatment centres, and unexpected side-effects may come out of the blue.
5. One factor which is becoming increasingly apparent is the need to monitor long-term consequences of treatment. A treatment or procedure introduced in good faith and with good results in a particular condition may, many years later, result in some unforeseen complication. The public need to recognize that such events can occur. In the search for new treatments, driven often by public demand, the long-term consequences need to be thought through, but even then may be unpredictable.

6. Miracle cures may occur, but by definition these are not routine events. So much of what is reported in the media raises expectation beyond what is reasonable or can be anticipated. Patients are often distraught when the evidence is placed before them, and seek other opinions and judgements.
7. The expectations raised are not only related to the doctor and the treatment, but to other members of the team, nurses, dieticians, pharmacists, and so on. Professionals are expected to provide a consistently high standard of service and, for almost all of the time, they do. But the professions need always to be aware of falling standards and take action.
8. In health issues, some of which have already been raised in the sections on perceptions of health, there is also sometimes a feeling that if someone would just *act*, the problem would go away. But again this denies the scientific uncertainty surrounding much of the research—whether it is about a drug, a chemical, an additive, or a food. There is thus a need to explore such issues of uncertainty with the public and assist in their understanding of health issues.
9. Research is at the heart of change and improving health and health care, but as noted earlier, there are problems, which need to be recognized. In the push for even better treatment, these must be remembered.

So what conclusions can be drawn from what at first sight may seem like a dispiriting list of arguments? Perhaps the most important is that we need to appreciate that patient expectations may change and that the professions need to respond to this in a positive way by, for example, improving services, better communication, and being 'customer' friendly. The corollary, however, is that patients and the public need to recognize the uncertainty of much of medicine and that it is an 'ART' as well as a 'SCIENCE', that ill health and ineffective therapies still exist, and that much remains to be discovered about improving health and health care.

5. Patient choice in health care

If we are serious about involving patients, then they need to have choice. This is not just about the doctor or nurse who will look after them, or the hospital to which they are to be referred, but choice about the kinds of treatment available. To do this they need information presented in a form which will encourage such choices to be made. For the professionals involved this can be a difficult process, particularly if the information is not black and white, and is complex to present. Hence the importance of communication skills. Perhaps more could be achieved in health by improving communication than almost any other factor. This includes communications between the professional and the patient, between professionals, and with the public. It is such an important subject that it is worth a short digression to deal with it at this stage.

Communication must be seen as a two-way process, and a means of opening channels and liberating action and choice. Communicating well means getting to know people and understanding them. It means sharing some of the pleasure and some of the pain. It means refocusing the traditional 'not getting involved mode' to getting involved without losing objectivity and professionalism. Martin Buber in his book *I and thou* describes the different nature of relationships between people as being of two kinds. The first is the relationship which is close (the 'I and thou' relationship) and which can result in a 'sharing of hearts'. Doctors or nurses who have had a close relationship with a patient who is dying will recognize this. There is no need to speak, all is understood. The second kind of relationship ('I and you') is of a more distant type and though it may be sufficient for some patients, perhaps it will not be enough for all. Communicating bad news is particularly difficult. Communication is of course not just about what is said, but what is done. Non-verbal communication is particularly powerful. Touch is such an important part of human communication, and can have a significant therapeutic effect if used with sensitivity.

Communication is also about seeing the patient through a crisis and helping them to benefit from their experience. Paul Tournier calls this 'creative suffering' and it is an essential aspect of patient care.

What needs to be recognized is that patients and their carers have enormous, if not unrivalled, experience of their condition or illness. When they wish to be involved then they can contribute not just to improving their own care but helping with others. The use of patient support groups, self-help groups, and information centres is a most helpful development and professionals have much to learn from them. Indeed it is a partnership concerned with the sharing of expertise and the widening of choice. In addition to providing someone to talk to who has been through the same illness, written information can be given and questions answered. The importance of advances in information technology mean that patients and the public have ready access to up-to-date information about disease and its treatment. Much of this is a normal part of good clinical practice, but it does not happen everywhere—to the detriment of patient care.

Communication skills are also about advocacy; of putting the needs of patients and the health needs of the public to the fore.

6. Public involvement in resource allocation and choices in health care

This is a most difficult topic and is currently at the forefront of discussion in most countries as they consider better ways of allocating resources. It should be clear, at the outset therefore, that there are no simple answers to the questions raised, and solutions will have to be found which try to reconcile different view points.

In essence the debate is between the rights of an individual to have treatment or care, no matter what the cost, against the common good and the most effective use of resources. In this context it is imperative that resources are not only considered as 'money' but as time and skills. These latter two may be more important than the cost of treatment. For example, if a doctor spends one hour with one patient, rather than 10 minutes, he cannot spend that time with another. Opportunity cost is important.

So there is a tension between the individual and the population and the question is how it can be resolved. It is likely that each individual case will be unique so what is required is a set of principles against which such cases can be judged. At the end of the day it will boil down to a judgement as to what is the most appropriate thing to do. Some of the principles involved, such as justice and equity, autonomy, and utility will be discussed in the next chapter in more detail, but it is useful to set them in the context of resource allocation. Finally, it should be noted that resources for health care (time, professional skills, and money) will always be limited and that this is not a new issue. What is new perhaps is the explicit discussion of the issue. Perhaps the most important principle in the debate is equity, by which is meant fairness and justice. Recent advances in medicine and changes in perception and expectations of patients and the public have highlighted this issue. It puts into perspective the tension between individual rights and the public good, and the effectiveness of the treatment.

For many conditions there are no particular problems. The condition is readily treated, the outcome is good, and the public good is enhanced. Coronary artery bypass surgery would be an example of this. Where it becomes more difficult is when it may become necessary to set limits, if any, to the number of such procedures or the outcomes carried out, and what the consequences would be for others who did not have coronary artery problems, but another disease, if all the resources were used for bypass surgery. It is also clear that some procedures are unproven, and of a research nature. It is essential that such research and development continues and that it is appropriately funded. But it is equally true that the wide dissemination and use of new treatments before evaluation would be a waste of resources, and might cause harm and distress to the patient. In between these two extremes of the well-established and effective therapy and the new development are a wide range of conditions and treatments which cannot be readily classified. This is seen in extreme form when an individual patient wishes a very expensive therapy, whose value is not proven or is considered to be of limited worth. In this instance the cost of treating one patient, within finite resources, is taken from another. And this is the nub of the debate.

Returning to a discussion of equity may help to clarify the issue, as there are two sides to the coin. The first is that there may be patients in the health care system (and this is not solely a UK issue) for whom treatment now would be of benefit and of proven value, but it is not available within existing resources. The second is the individual patient who wishes treatment at whatever the cost, for a small chance of success—thus denying treatment to others. It should be emphasized again that this effect is likely to be independent of the level of funding, unless that funding was infinite. In the real world there will always be finite resources, and such instances are likely to occur with increasing frequency.

The question for society, therefore, is to consider the fairness of the allocation of resources for any particular form of therapy and begin to set a framework which could be agreed across the population as a whole. The well-known initiative in Oregon, where the population were involved in setting priorities, has shown how difficult this can be, and it is not the only way forward. At the end of the day it will be a matter of judgement about the fairness of allocating resources, and common sense will need to be one of the values which will determine such choices.

7. Risk communication

Almost all public figures who have an interest in health (politicians, professionals, and managers) will, at some time or another, have to speak to the public about a health matter. This might be related to the health service or to a public health topic. The major issue generally boils down to a consideration of uncertainty and to translating complex scientific issues into words and actions which are understandable. Risk communication is the art of making such connections, and there is already considerable literature on the subject.

There are four major factors to be considered before looking at some of the ways of improving communication. The first, and most obvious, is that of the characteristics of the scientific information and its limitations. Inevitably it is complex and normally surrounded by uncertainties and caveats. The second is that of the person communicating the information. For example, the lack of trust in the individual by the public, his or her own skills and training in communication, and often the difficulty of dealing with different agencies, all of whom give different messages. The third is that of the demands of the media. They need information, they have tight deadlines, and they generally wish to develop a story with a 'human' angle. Finally there is the public itself. Scientific knowledge, the ability to understand complex issues, the use of statistics, are all less well developed than they might be—hence the importance of initiatives such as the public understanding of science. Communication also emphasizes the need for the language of health, of health literacy, to be more readily understood in order that the public at large can have an important part in the debate.

With this as a background, how can risk communication be improved? First it is necessary to define the aim of the topic. The purpose of risk communication is *not* to defuse public concern or avoid action, but to produce an informed public that is involved, reasonable, thoughtful, and collaborative. The quotation at the start of this chapter says this more elegantly. First, we need to accept and ensure that the public are seen as legitimate partners in the debate and seek ways to involve them. Secondly, there is a need to listen carefully and be open and frank about the issue in question. Thirdly, is the need to co-ordinate all participating agencies and ensure that the media are also seen as partners.

However, the most important issue is the development of trust and credibility of the individual giving the information. He or she should be a good communicator, with competence and experience, who shows interest and concern in the issue. Judgement by the public about the credibility of the source is made within a few minutes and unless this trust can be established rapidly then the involvement and debate may get off to a bad start. Organizations, such as health authorities and hospitals, should therefore plan ahead for such eventualities and ensure that those who speak have the right characteristics and background.

At the end of the day it is the public who need to know about the issues and make up their minds. Involvement and participation are the heart of the process of risk communication.

A case study in cancer and the language of risk

Of all the diseases in the Western world, cancer is perhaps the most alarming. It is an enigma, and in spite of a remarkable number of advances in the understanding of the disease and in the treatment of specific types of cancer, much still remains to be learned. As a group of diseases, the cancers are of interest not only to the scientific and medical community, but to the public and politicians. Rarely a day goes by without some new breakthrough in cancer treatment, or in the identification of another substance or environmental factor which might cause cancer. One of the key issues surrounding cancer is the assessment of risk, both from environmental factors, and from clinical treatment, and how that is communicated to the public. The need for adequate data is therefore clear, and is the foundation for appropriate clinical and public health practice. In this regard cancer can be used as a model for a variety of other diseases and, as the database is generally better in cancer than elsewhere, provides examples of how some of the principles involved in the control of a disease can be put into practice. Thus a consideration of cancer can be used as a case study from which general lessons may be learned.

Assumptions

There are two assumptions. The first is that there is a requirement to assess the needs of the country and that population-based cancer registration has value and is probably better than other disease-based databases. The second is that the public have a right to information and to be involved in the choice of treatment. In examining the first of these assumptions—the value of cancer registration—there is clearly a benefit in the assessment and planning of population needs, in carrying out epidemiological studies and in performing risk assessment. It is also of great value in evaluating the outcome of treatment options, and in the identification of basic research relating to the pathogenesis of individual cancers. Linked to geographical information systems, cancer registration can provide a remarkable range of information at a series of different population levels. However, it is not without its problems. Incomplete and inadequate data are perhaps the greatest of these. When particular cancers have a low incidence, or the numbers are small, then it is often difficult to make links between particular factors and the cancers themselves. In addition to this, while correlations may be identified, establishing a plausible hypothesis and testing it is often much more difficult. These conclusions are equally relevant to other illnesses.

It is also a fair assumption that the public should be involved in the understanding of why cancers are caused and to be encouraged to avoid risks of developing cancer. In addition to this, where a variety of different treatments are available, the use of registration data in identifying best practice can inform individual patients and allow them to have an appropriate choice over the method of treatment which best suits them. The main problem, however, is perhaps the uncertainty arising from lack of data available, and the difficulties of making a full risk assessment. While individuals may be able to avoid some risk factors, they may not be able to avoid others which may seem to be imposed on them. Thus, simply the identification of a risk factor may not be sufficient. However, the assumption still holds that public involvement is central.

The role of cancer registration in the assessment of risks and benefits

There are multiple examples of the identification by epidemiological techniques of factors associated with a higher incidence of cancer. The most obvious ones are cigarette smoking and lung cancer, radiation and skin cancer, high-risk sexual behaviour and cervical cancer, genetic implications of cancer, Burkitts lymphoma, radon, dioxins, and a whole range of occupational cancers. These make it clear that under some circumstances it is possible to identify and to quantify the risks and, where appropriate, for these risks to be avoided or removed.

Cancer registration also permits better recognition of treatment options. Using controlled clinical trials, best practice can be identified. Staging in prognostic factors can also be identified and allow better stratification and more accurate assessment of outcomes. Of particular interest is the relationship between the specialist treatment centre and the generalist treatment centre. This is an important debate which is ongoing at the present time. And lastly, there is the issue of the publication of outcomes for the benefit of the public and of individual patients. These are clearly vital matters which relate directly to the quality of the evidence available.

This leads to the next major issue, which is the problem of certainty in science. For each of the factors mentioned, and for some issues to be discussed later, there are limits to the confidence in the data. In some instances, when probed by the question 'How sure are you of the data?', the epidemiologist has to hedge the outcomes with a variety of different caveats. This significantly weakens the case and can make it difficult to set public policy.

The problem for decision makers is not when the evidence is clear, but when it is weak or incomplete, or even at the stage of a hypothesis. In this instance, they have two courses of action: one, to go beyond the evidence and act in a precautionary manner; or two, to wait until the evidence becomes clear, which may take years or even decades. There needs therefore to be a judgement about the quality of the evidence, and of the implications of acting on that evidence. This requires openness and sharing of information. A third compromise option may be possible in some circumstances. Some examples can highlight this. There have been a number of studies which relate diet to the development of specific cancers. However, close examination of the data shows that in many instances this is not quite as clear and obvious as it might seem. Another example would be the possibility of non-ionizing radiation causing some forms of cancer. The data in this area is weak and a plausible hypothesis linking non-ionizing radiation and cancer is not clear but has been suggested in some studies. A third example is the use of small-area statistics in the identification of a link between a point source of an environmental hazard and the development of a specific cancer. Whilst the technology has advanced considerably, there are still a number of major uncertainties. Finally, the treatment of breast cancer can be considered. This is one of the most intensively studied diseases across the developing world. In spite of this there are still significant areas of debate about best management and in how to advise patients.

The relationship between the science base, the knowledge available, the evidence accumulated, and the public policy which derives from them is one of the major issues for those who make decisions about public health. Such decisions can be extraordinarily difficult, and the costs of taking action based on minimal evidence or simply on the basis of an hypothesis can be very considerable indeed. Thus, epidemiological techniques, and the data generated from cancer registration are very powerful in identifying correlations between diseases and clinical outcomes. However, they do have limitations in setting public policy.

The importance of assessing risk

The discussion so far has been based on the assumption that the identification of a risk factor which involves an individual changing behaviour is straightforward and clear. However, this is generally not the case. How people perceive health issues and risk, and how they make choices about their own behaviour, does not always fall into a rational pattern.

Before discussing this further a few definitions may be helpful. First, a **hazard** is set of circumstances which may have harmful consequences. The **probability** of a **hazard** causing such effects is the **risk** of the adverse event occurring. A **hazard** is therefore a **potential** risk and does not indicate whether the event will occur to a particular individual. However, it should be clear that adverse events can and do occur. Infections, environmental hazards, procedures, treatments, and investigations all carry both risks and benefits. It is the individual's perception of these risks and benefits which is perhaps crucial.

Take the issue of cigarette smoking. The risk is clearly established and well-known, yet 30 per cent of the adult population continue to smoke. In this instance the value of smoking is seen, to the individual, to be greater than the value of not smoking. The fact that cigarette smoking is an addictive behavioural pattern is no doubt a partial explanation. However, over the last few years, a wide variety of 'health scares' have shown that the public can very rapidly change their behaviour, despite evidence which is often quite weak. Although the risk of a hazard occurring may well be very small, individuals may choose **not** to take even such a small risk, and therefore avoid it.

There is an important distinction to be made between absolute and relative risk. This is best exemplified in relation to oral contraceptives, and the risk of venous thrombosis by third generation contraceptive pills. It is true that the relative risk of venous thrombosis (defined as venous thrombotic episodes (VTEs)) is doubled with the new pills compared with second generation ones. However, the absolute risk is negligible for both types of pills, and is much smaller than the risk through pregnancy. The public presentation of these figures cause great anxiety, yet the increase of risk is very small indeed (Table 4.1). The message to continue to take the pill seemed to be ignored.

There is a further concern on the possibility of unknown or unpredicted side-effects. These may happen many years after the treatment or exposure, and may affect all or only a small proportion of those treated or exposed. This is the nature of the development of new treatments or investigations. Their immediate benefit may be great or indeed may be demanded by the public, only later to realize that the long-term consequences may be adverse. Science is expected to deliver. But the public need to understand more about the nature of science and the real differences of opinion which may occur during the often unstructured process of discovery.

In clinical terms, the risk benefit analysis is similar. For example, it may be that the patient has a 1 in 100 chance of benefiting from a particular form of treatment, and they opt to take that chance. It is also possible however that 99 patients will have ineffective treatment, and treatment which may indeed lead to serious side-effects.

Thus, in understanding issues surrounding risk assessment, perception is a key element in patient and public choice. Information sharing is critical. Cancer provides a good model of how such issues can be debated and general principles derived.

Table 4.1—Comparative risks of venous thrombotic episodes (VTEs)

	VTE per 100 000 women / year	Mortality per one million women / year
No use of pill	5	0.5
Pill	15	1.5
Low-dose pill	30	3.0
Pregnancy	60	6.0

The language of risk

How then can risks be described, and what does the language mean? Risks in recent years have been talked about in a variety of ways, such as negligible, minimal, remote, very small, small, and so on. The public and professionals are rightly confused by such a range of words. A classification is required to assist in the understanding of the process, but in doing so such terms need to be qualified by other words which may be equally important. These include:

1. **Avoidable—unavoidable**
This is an important distinction and can radically shift the perception of risk. This allows the individual to exercise choice, and for the public to be involved in the decision-making process.
2. **Justifiable—unjustifiable**
These words carry values with them, and risks may be taken in some instances but not others. For example, the use of a drug, with known side-effects, to treat a particular condition, may be justifiable to achieve some benefit. However, if the patient was pregnant this might not be considered justifiable.
3. **Acceptable—unacceptable**
Once again these are value-laden words, but need to be used in particular contexts. In general, an unacceptable risk would not be tolerated except for special reasons in exceptional circumstances, for example, in the use of an unproven method of treatment as a therapy of last resort.
4. **Serious—non-serious**
These again are words which refer to particular situations but, in this instance, they refer to risks which are life threatening or likely to cause disability or morbidity. In the case of clinical conditions they need to be put in the context of the diagnosis which may be minor or life threatening. In the presentation of risk, the seriousness of the problem needs to be taken into account as well as the frequency.

Central to these provisos is the risk benefit analysis and how this is perceived by individuals. Some may not wish to take any risks in spite of the possibility of real benefit. Others will take a chance even when the benefit is likely to be very low. With these provisos in mind the following classification might be used. It draws on a great deal of other work and is an attempt to answer the public's questions as to what is meant by 'safe'. This classification is relevant only in relation to the description of risk, and not in relation to how that risk might be managed. It is put forward for debate and is not meant to be a definitive classification:

1. **Negligible**
This would describe an adverse event occurring at less than one per million and, if of an environmental nature, or the consequence of a health care intervention, would have little impact on everyday living. It should be noted however that this does not mean that the event is not important—it almost certainly will be to the individual concerned—nor that it is not possible to reduce the risk even further. Other words which can be used in this context are 'remote' or 'insignificant'. If the word 'safe' is to be used it must be seen to mean negligible but should **not** imply no or zero risk.
2. **Minimal**
This would mean that the risk was in the range of between one in a million and 1 in 100 000 of a serious event occurring, and that the conduct of normal life is not generally affected as long as reasonable precautions are taken. The possibility of a risk is thus clearly noted and could be described as 'acceptable'—a word which might also be used as an alternative, as could 'very small'. What is of course acceptable to one person may not be to another.
3. **Very low**
This would describe a risk of between 1 in 100 000 and 1 in 10 000, and thus begins to describe an event or a consequence of a health care procedure becoming more frequent.

4. **Low**
This would relate to a risk which was between 1 in 10 000 and 1 in 1000. Once again, this would apply to many clinical procedures and environmental hazards. Other words which might be used include 'reasonable', 'tolerable', and 'small'. Many risks fall into this very broad category.
5. **Moderate**
This would cover a risk of between 1 in 1000 and 1 in 100, and include a wide range of procedures, treatments, and environmental events.
6. **High**
These become fairly regular events and would occur at a rate greater than 1 in 100. They might also be described as 'frequent', 'significant', or 'serious'.
7. **Unknown risk**
This circumstance occurs when the level of risk is unknown or unquantifiable. This is not uncommon in the early stages of an environmental event or the start of a newly recognized disease process. The beginning of the HIV epidemic would be an example of this.

Which of these terms apply to the individual case is of course a matter of discussion and debate. They may vary from time to time, with changing circumstances and information on the level of risk. It is possible, for example, for new research and knowledge to alter the level of risk—either way. Similarly, how it is presented is important. For example, the level of risk for smoking cigarettes could be recorded as low if it is measured as the risk of dying in one year from smoking 10 cigarettes a day. The lifetime risk of dying however is between 1:2 and 1:5, and this would therefore place it in the high-risk category.

The use of these terms is further described in Table 4.2, in relation to a range of different risks—some familiar, some less so.

The foregoing discussion leads naturally to a consideration of how best to communicate the level of risk associated with a particular health or health care issue to the public. The media have a very important responsibility in

Table 4.2—Risk of an individual dying in any one year or developing an adverse response

Term used	Risk estimate	Example	
High	Greater than 1:100	(A) Transmission to susceptible household contacts of measles and chickenpox[5]	1:1–1:2
		(A) Transmission of HIV from mother to child (Europe)[2]	1:6
		(A) GI effects of antibiotics[4]	1:10–1:20
Moderate	Between 1:100–1:1000	(D) All natural causes, age 40[1]	1:850
Low	Between 1:1000–1:10 000	(D) All kinds of violence and poisoning[1]	1:3300
		(D) Influenza[8]	1:5000
		(D) Accident on road[1]	1:8000
Very low	Between 1:1000–1:100 000	(D) Leukaemia[1]	1:12 000
		(D) Playing soccer[1]	1:25 000
		(D) Accident at home[1]	1:26 000
		(D) Accident at work[1]	1:43 000
		(D) Homicide[1]	1:100 000
Minimal	Between 1:100 000–1:1 000 000	(D) Accident on railway[1]	1:500 000
		(A) Vaccination associated polio[3]	1:1 000 000
Negligible	Less than 1:1 000 000	(D) Hit by lightning[1]	1:10 000 000
		(D) Release of radiation by nuclear power station[1]	1:10 000 000

References

1. (1990). *The BMA guide to living with risk.* Penguin Books
2. Peckham, C. and Gibb, D. (1995). *New Eng J Med.*, **333**, 298–302.
3. (1992). *Immunisation against infectious disease.* HMSO, London.
4. Ness *et al.* (1993). *J Chemotherapy*, **5**, 67–93.
5. (1975). *Harrison's principles of internal medicine*, 9th edn, p. 793.

Key

(D) Dying
(A) Adverse response

this regard. A number of guidelines have been described and they include: the importance of credible sources of advice; openness; sharing uncertainty; the need to accept the public as partners; careful planning; listening to concerns; co-ordinating with other credible sources; and meeting the needs of the media.

It is hoped that this preliminary classification of the terminology relating to risk is of value, and that it will be the subject of further debate. However, it does emphasize the importance of ensuring that the public are full partners in the process of risk assessment and management, and it is only with such involvement that progress can be made.

The value of the science base and the knowledge base is clear, but unanswered questions remain, and there is often real uncertainty within science itself. This makes it difficult to present the public with clear information in all instances. As far as they are concerned, they have a right to as much information as is available, but they also have to appreciate that this information may not be complete, and that it may not be possible to provide further information on a particular issue without more work, resources, and, in particular, time. However, this does emphasize the need for an individual's choice and the importance of their perception of risk. From a public point of view, these should be, wherever possible, evidence based. However, when there is uncertainty, the need to take precautionary action, or to wait and see, is an extremely difficult decision requiring judgement and the participation of the public.

In summary, therefore, if the maximum benefit is to be gained from the collection and the analysis of data, the public must be seen as full partners in the process, but they must also recognize that the uncertainty of science remains a significant issue.

8. The role of the media in health

The media have an important role in shaping our views on health. Printed, audio, and visual media can influence huge numbers of people, and change attitudes and opinions. It is for this reason that the media are of considerable value to those wishing to improve health. Almost every day there is a health or health care story which catches the headlines. This ability to influence carries with it responsibilities to get the facts right and to present a balanced picture. It is particularly easy to be destructive: the formula is simple. First select any disease. Identify a few patients who have had a bad experience, a professor who has unconventional views, and another who is just about to publish a new finding, and the programme is almost made. Add to this a government official who is not privy to such information and you have all the ingredients for confrontation and, in some cases, confusion of the public. The need for good and unhindered journalism is clear, but the effects of poor journalism on the public are less certain. Attitudes to food, lifestyle, and behaviour can be rapidly altered—if the 'salmonella and eggs' incident is anything to go by. Bad news is often good news for the media, but the good news about health is often neglected. Public expectations are often raised by stories in the media about successful treatment or new research. Scare stories, miracle cures, and environmental risks can set the agenda and change public perceptions.

Anyone with an interest in changing health must therefore spend time with the media, be prepared to help, and to recognize the constraints they are under. Journalists can be of enormous value if their skills are harnessed to improve health and inform the public.

9. The public and their role in medical research and professional education

First, professional education. How professionals are educated is of considerable interest to patients and the public. After all, patients are at the centre of the care process, and thus should be the focus of professional education. Is medical education, for example, too important to be left to doctors, and nurse education to nurses? As has been said already in this chapter, health professionals are also citizens who happen to have specialized knowledge. How much more competent to judge the balance of medical education and its curriculum would a lawyer be, or the manager of a supermarket, or a young mother, or the secretary of a disease-specific patient group? Their input may be valuable on the technical side of education, though this may not always be the case. They are more likely to have a vital contribution on attitudes and behaviour, and on what is often known as the 'bedside manner'. This should certainly ensure that change occurs both in the content and method of teaching. Many of the important innovations in medical education occurring in this country reflect these views. While patients may not find it easy to comment on technical issues, they can certainly have a view on the subjects in the curriculum. Increasing concern about ethical issues, communication skills, public health, and community issues could be part of this. The General Medical Council (GMC), in its recent document *Tomorrow's Doctors*, tackles many of these issues—and 25 per cent of its membership is non-medical.

Public and patient involvement in research is a fascinating issue. From the point of view of the patient, the issue is essentially one of consent. There are so many words related to consent that it is difficult to discuss them all—implied, explicit, informed, written, verbal, are all words which are used. What the patient probably wants is an explanation of the procedure, its likely consequences and outcomes, the other treatments which are available, and the implications of not being treated. All of this to be given in an intelligible manner, with time and the opportunities to ask questions. This process is relevant not only to new and innovative procedures, but to well-established ones.

The second area of public involvement is on research ethics committees. These are set up to review, not the science of new procedures, though this is relevant, but the ethical implications for the patient, before the doctor or nurse can progress the trial of a new treatment or investigation. This is a very important process and those representing the public have a great responsibility. But how should they be chosen? Do they need to be lawyers, or moral philosophers, or will any member of the public do? Around the country different models of ethics committees are being developed and their experience will help to inform the others. This is an example where the need to get started has allowed good practice to be developed and the expertise to be developed and shared.

10. The public understanding of health, science, and medicine

While professional groups have a responsibility to make information available to the public in an easily assimilable way, so the public too have a responsibility. The world of science and medicine is changing fast. New technology will bring new opportunities and new problems. The public, and with them decision makers who have no medical or scientific background, should see it as part of their broader education to keep well informed.

11. Conclusions

This chapter set out to highlight and clarify some of the ways in which the public can become increasingly involved in health and health care. It also tries to underline some of the tensions including perceptions of health and expectations of improving health and health care. The discussion about how best to bring together professional views, patient expectations, rights of the patient, and the public good is now well under way, and to be welcomed. The potential for health will only be achieved if the energy of patients and the population is appropriately harnessed.

Further reading

BMA. (1990). *The BMA guide to living with risk.* Penguin Books.
Martin Buber, (1958). *I and thou.* SCM Press, Edinburgh.
Paul Tournier, *Creative suffering.* SCM Press, Edinburgh.
The Royal Society. (1993). *Risk: analysis, preception and management.*

5

Ethical issues in public health

1. Introduction

Ethical issues are at the heart of the practice of public health, and central to the day-to-day work of those involved in improving health. They were raised as one of the basic principles at the start of this book. In considering such issues, two broad concepts are brought together. The first is how we manage risk and uncertainty. If we knew for certain that a particular procedure (such as a medical treatment) always produced a particular outcome (such as cure), then the need to consider the ethical implications would be less, as the uncertainty would be removed. Or if we knew that exposure to a chemical would always result in an illness, or exposure to a bacterium or virus always resulted in clinical infection, then the matter would be simpler. A consideration of ethical issues helps us see our way through such uncertainties. Similarly when such problems concern the public, and affect the population as a whole, the way in which they are communicated must reflect this uncertainty of risk. (This has already been discussed in Chapter 4). The second concept is that of the value base from which such judgements are made. This is perhaps the most difficult part as without an understanding of the values of society, culture, populations, groups, it becomes very difficult to interpret decisions affecting health policy. For example, a society which has the importance of the family as one of its main values will consider issues of health differently from one in which the basic unit is the individual.

This chapter first considers the role of ethics and the value base from which judgements are made. These should be viewed in the light of the definition of health and its determinants in Chapter 1. This then leads to a discussion on some of the principles involved, illustrated with hypothetical examples which highlight some of the practical issues. The aim is to show that there is generally no single answer and that decisions have to be made on the basis of judgements. For a longer discussion on these topics the reader is referred to *Healthy Respect* by Downie and Calman, and *Health promotion* by Downie, Tannahill, and Tannahill.

2. The ethical base

The role of ethics is to clarify thinking and to assist in the analysis of a particular problem. It is about trying to make decision making more rational and to manage uncertainty. The key issue for public health is the balance of the rights of the individual with those of the community or the population as a whole. This is equally applicable in the control of a particular disease (for example, isolation for an infection) or the availability of a treatment (for example, heart transplantation) to some or all members of the public. Decisions in these areas are very difficult to make but are at the heart of the matter. The role of ethics is to provide a framework which will reduce, but not eliminate, the uncertainty in decision making. At the end of the day judgement will still be required.

Such issues are not new and, in one form or another, have been around for centuries. Hippocratic writings comment on such topics and over the years publications, declarations, and Acts of Parliament have been developed to deal with specific issues and to codify, regulate, and interpret the will of the people. The introduction of seat belt legislation, or the use of crash helmets, limit an individual's liberties, but are in the interests of the public good. In recent years the advances made in medicine, the changing demographic picture, and greater openness in public decision making have all highlighted the need for public debate, and this is taken up in Chapter 4. The subject is not confined to this country. Indeed it would be difficult to consider ethical issues in public health without mentioning some of the international problems. Matters of starvation, war, and the environment all have an international dimension and an impact on health. Ethical issues are of such importance that the European Region of WHO now has one of its 38 targets specifically related to ethics. This chapter will deal mainly with issues relevant to this country, and Chapter 9 will pick up those with a particular international flavour. Further discussion of ethical issues related to health care are considered in Chapter 10, and to professional roles in Chapter 12.

3. The value base

Almost all that is relevant to the practice of public health, other than the knowledge base, are the values upon which decisions are made—basic human values; public and societal values; political, professional, and educational values. Associated with this are the questions 'Where do values come from?' and 'How are values determined?'. Each category of values will now be examined in turn.

1. Basic human values

Five basic human values can be identified with particular relevance to health and health care: autonomy, justice, beneficence, non-malevolence, and utility. In rather simpler language: the rights of the individual, fairness and equity, doing good—not doing harm, and the common good—or the greatest good for the greatest number. Each of these is important, but may be in conflict with the others. For example, as part of a treatment, the doctor may need to cause pain to do good. However, the key conflict is the relationship between the rights of the individual (autonomy), and utility and justice: the individual versus the population. In the examples which follow this will be the principal issue raised. For example, how does one deal with high-cost treatment which will benefit only a limited number of people compared to the many who might benefit if the funding was used for other, equally valid, purposes. It challenges the way in which resources are allocated.

2. Societal and political values

A wide range of issues could be included under this heading. Cultural values in relation to women or homosexuals would be examples of this. Political values determine the policy decisions on such topics as the structure and organization of the health care system, and the wide variety of such systems throughout the world illustrate this. In this country health is of importance to every political party and all recognize this in their manifestos. Values in society shape our decisions and judgements, and they are constantly changing. For example, the way in which society initially responded to the HIV epidemic was narrowly focused on 'gay issues' and was seen as 'something to do with them'. The rise of numbers in the heterosexual population with HIV infection and its emergence as a huge worldwide problem has shifted attitudes, and this is a good example of 'evolutionary ethics'. The legal system is also in constant movement, redefining concepts and reinterpretating the law in response to changing attitudes. The debate on child protection would be an example of this.

3. Personal values

What determines personal values? Relevant factors include upbringing, education, peer pressure, personal experience, religion, culture, and special knowledge (such as being a doctor or nurse). Is it or is it not relevant to have a medical degree to make difficult decisions and judgements about health care? It may not make it any easier but it should not make it worse, and doctors are after all citizens like everyone else. It is not difficult to think of examples in private life to show how values and choices are shaped and altered. How you choose your food, your friends, or your taste in music make you realize how much your values have been influenced by past and current experience, friends, and values within society. The importance of this section is to emphasize that choices and values are often founded, not on the knowledge base, but on contacts and conversations with those we trust and believe. The power of the story, or anecdote, is very strong indeed, and may override the factual information available to us. The irrational may easily bypass the rational.

4. *Professional values*

How do these relate to personal values? For example, in relation to smoking, alcohol, exercise? What additional responsibilities, if any, do health care professionals have in these areas? Professional values are at the core of declarations and oaths which have been extant for many years. It is important to examine whether or not they conflict with societal or political values. These are discussed more fully later on.

5. *Educational values*

It is sometimes forgotten that there is a 'hidden curriculum' in professional education which sends messages to students and others about how patients should be treated and resources used. This value base is established early on and should be taken into account in any description of professional values. It reinforces the importance of the teacher and the educational institution in establishing the ethical base of medical practice.

4. Equity and equality

These concepts have been discussed in detail in Chapter 2. Suffice it to say that they are fundamental to the value base.

The variations in health which exist in all countries and in all towns and cities are the clearest evidence of inequalities in health. Problems of poverty, deprivation, and alienation are at the heart of this. In the words of the old ballad:

> It's the same the whole world over
> It's the poor what gets the blame.
> It's the rich what get the pleasure
> Ain't it all a blooming shame.

Poverty is not inevitable, but there are no simple solutions to the problems. The most vulnerable in society need help and support if we are to achieve 'health for all'.

5. Some general issues

In the earlier part of the chapter it was noted that the practice of public health depended on the knowledge base and the values of society. Within that discussion the issue of the definition of health and its determinants, as discussed in Chapter 1, are very relevant. This includes the fact that health itself is an important human value. However, any review of ethical issues in public health has to recognize a number of difficulties, which include:

1. Most problems are complex and there may not be a 'right' answer.
2. Choices have to be made within defined limits and constraints.
3. The knowledge base is one component of decision making—but *only* one.
4. Logical argument and analysis are only one part of the process. Those who put together a clear, well worked-out case and a rational statement to be presented to a decision-making body, will realize the truth of this. This is part of learning how decisions are made.
5. The public dimension in decision making needs to be considered. Who are they, and how do they become involved?

6. No matter how straightforward the issues may seem, there will always be room for differences of view. Within the public health team these differences may be very important and they have to be recognized and dealt with.
7. Information will become increasingly available which will show variations in health and the outcome of health care in different populations and in different parts of the country. Such information will raise major ethical issues both for individuals and communities. This will test the value base of society and decisions about the targeting of resources and the principle of equity. This is very much in line with the 'Our Healthier Nation' in which key areas set the agenda (see Chapter 3). Through healthy alliances, groups, and settings, energy is directed to change targeted specifically at these key topics.

At this stage two conclusions can be drawn. First, that values are complex but important in decision making, and a knowledge of how values are derived can be useful in the process. Second, that health is an important human value. Choices about health and health care are determined in part by the knowledge base, but also in part by the values of society, these being represented through duly elected representatives in government. An interesting analysis of some of these issues has been written by Hans Kung in his book *Global responsibility. In search of a new world ethic.* More recently, J. K. Galbraith has written *The good society,* which also takes up these issues. Interestingly *Sybil*, written by Benjamin Disraeli in the nineteenth century, comes to many of the same conclusions. In all of this of course the importance of common sense must not be underrated.

6. Some examples

In this final section some specific case studies will be examined. These are hypothetical, rather than live issues, in order to focus the discussion on principles rather than details:

1. A new virus is discovered which causes a fatal heart disease. It will cost £3 million per year to screen blood for transfusion, and there are around 750 000 transfusions in England each year. Having piloted the test in a series of donors it is found to be present in either 1:1000, 1:100 000, 1 in a million, or 1 in 10 million. If the figure was 1 in a million, then each life saved would cost £2–3 million pounds. The figures are those of 1994, and from past experience are considered realistic. The question is at what level you would consider it worthwhile to introduce the test? A related issue, of course, is who should make the decision?

This specific example raises a second point—that of communicating the risk to the public, having made the decision. For example, if it was decided *not* to test at the level of 1:100 000 how would this be discussed with the public, and how would the decision be justified?

2. One of the most exciting areas of human biology is the increasing understanding of the human genome and how it works. Already limited genetic engineering procedures in humans can be carried out and, within a few years, more will be feasible. It will become possible to analyze the genetic background of an individual and identify potential susceptibility to disease. Under these circumstances, whose information is this, and who can have access to it? Many more such questions will be raised in the future.

3. A new treatment becomes available for lung cancer. The drug costs about £5000 per course of treatment. It cures about 25 per cent of patients, a further 25 per cent are improved, thus leaving 50 per cent who show no benefit. It causes around 0.1 per cent of patients to develop leukaemia in the long term, and there is 1 per cent acute mortality. The drug has to be given in special centres and in-patient treatment costs £10 000 per patient, in addition to drug costs. There are around 32 000 new cases of lung cancer each year in England. The total cost if each patient were to be treated would be £480 million. Pressure groups are saying that patients are dying, and there is great pressure to introduce the treatment. If all patients with lung cancer were to be treated with the new drug then the cost per cure would

be £60 000. A decision will have to be made soon, what will it be?

4. A common, and generally beneficial drug treatment for a chronic disease has been used for many years. A new diagnostic test is introduced which picks up a low, but measurable, level of renal damage in patients given the drug. A decision has to be made as to whether or not the treatment is withdrawn. This raises an important issue which has already surfaced in other areas—that of the introduction of increasingly sophisticated monitoring procedures after the intervention is in routine use. This is likely to become more common. Procedures which were considered to be safe and effective turn out to have problems. In instances such as these how is the public to be informed and assisted in decision making? They have a right as citizens to the information.

Each of these hypothetical examples raises the importance of the outcome of health and health care, and indicates the extent of the problem.

7. Some conclusions

Ethical issues are complex and associated with risk and uncertainty. In making decisions values are important, but they also have to be realistic. This means that the public should be involved in decision making and have ownership of the decisions. In some instances a 'don't know' response may be indicated and acceptable. In each case judgements have to be made, wherever possible, on a knowledge of outcomes, and the consequences of the actions and decisions must be considered and thought through.

For the future, several issues need to be emphasized. First, the need for greater public involvement. Second, the need for better information on outcomes to reduce uncertainty, whether related to health or health care. Lastly, as a consequence of this, better professional education is required to ensure that these issues are raised and discussed. The value base of professional practice needs constantly to be tested and reviewed.

Teaching and learning about medical ethics

The subject cannot simply be taught or learned in an abstract way, by reading texts by experts. It requires some practical examples to bring to life the complex issues involved. Ethics is a practical subject. It also requires the facility to discuss one's own views with others. There will be differences of view, and these do need to be taken into account. Learning to work with a colleague who has different opinions about health or health care can be challenging. However, it is the real world. There are many ways of sharing views—notably by group discussion centred on particular problems. Another way of looking at the issues is through the eyes of artists and writers. Such people can illuminate human feelings and values. The next chapter shows how this approach, that of using the creative arts, can be of value to patients as well as professionals.

Further reading

Downie, R. S. and Calman, K. C. (1995). *Healthy Respect*, 2nd edn. Oxford University Press.

Downie, R. S., Tannahill, D. and Tannahill, C. (1995). *Health Promotion*, 2nd edn. Oxford University Press.

Kung, H. (1990). *Global responsibility: in search of a new world ethic.* SCM Press Ltd, Edinburgh.

Galbraith, J. K. (1996). *The good society: the humane agenda.* Sinclair-Stevenson, London.

Disraeli, B. *Sybil.* Penguin Books.

6

The humanities in clinical practice

The humanities may be defined broadly to include literature, art, music, ethics, and philosophy. Why is it important to discuss a topic like the humanities in clinical practice, and what relevance does it have to the practice of modern medicine or management? In fact, they bring a different dimension to clinical practice as, in addition to considering the *science* of healing, the humanities make us more aware of the importance of the *art* of healing. One aspect of the humanities is in their relevance to the ethical base of clinical practice. There are many reasons why an understanding of ethical issues is important: it enables us to clarify our thinking, to assist in analysis and decision making, and to help to manage uncertainty. Dealing with uncertainty is a very real problem—in treating individual patients; in how an organization, whether a hospital trust or a health authority, will respond to a particular problem; and of course, in how the public should be involved in such important issues.

Important ethical principles including justice (fairness), individual rights (autonomy), doing good (beneficence), not doing harm (non-malevolence), and utility have already been described in Chapter 5. It is very clear that at times there is great conflict between these principles, particularly between autonomy and utility. Recent examples have shown how, both at a patient and a health authority level, these differences may not only become highly public, but are matters of real uncertainty and judgement. One way to approach this of course is to use the 'my mother' principle. If it was your mother, your child, or your loved one, what in fact would you wish to do? This becomes even more relevant when issues concerning quality of life are considered. Quality of life is an important issue but an extremely difficult one to define. The holistic nature of care, therefore, must always be considered. Such basic human ethical principles and values are at the heart of clinical care.

But where do values come from? Values come from basic human instincts, through personal development, contacts and experiences, from society itself. Superimposed on these are important professional values. The doctor, the nurse, or the health service manager has brought together these values in a personal way, and it is these experiences which enable him or her to make decisions in times of uncertainty. What is important however is that such personal values are tested against others, and that the individual is able both to justify a particular course of action, as required, and to recognize that others may also have legitimate views which may be different from theirs.

Consideration of the role of the humanities begins with the problem of knowledge, and the fact that knowledge cannot be compartmentalized. To be an effective health professional requires knowledge not only of one's own specialism but of related subjects and, beyond that, of wider experiences such as those to do with ethics and philosophy and the humanities in general. What then is the role of the humanities? This Chapter will identify a few of the issues which may be relevant.

1. Literature and medicine

The first issue relates to literature and medicine and builds on a series of personal experiences which have shown the value of such cross-discipline initiatives.[1,2,3,4] During a series of courses with medical students and nurses, a whole range of books, poems, and plays were discussed, including Chekov's story, '*Ward 6*', which describes how a doctor working in a Russian community hospital for psychiatric patients befriends one of the patients, and is eventually admitted to the hospital. It illustrates very clearly the boundaries between normality and abnormality. Another important work used was *'The cocktail party'* by T. S. Eliot. During the first act of this play there is plenty of talk at the cocktail party, but no listening. For a fourth-year student to comment that this is sometimes the situation between doctors and patients shows an enormous sense of maturity and understanding of the process of medical care. If you wish to have an understanding of tuberculosis from a patient perspective, then Thomas Mann's book *The magic mountain* is remarkable. The play written by Brian Clarke, *'Whose life is it anyway'*, highlights many current issues and dilemmas relevant to terminating life. Consider this dialogue between two doctors, in a scene from the play:

Dr Scott: But surely a wish to die is not necessarily a symptom of insanity? A man might want to die for perfectly sane reasons.

Dr Emerson: No Claire, a doctor can't accept choice for death. He is committed to life. When a patient is brought into my unit he is in a bad way. I don't stand about thinking whether or not it is worth saving his life, I haven't the time for doubts, I get in there, do whatever I can to save life. I am doctor, not a judge.

Dr Scott: I hope you will forgive me Sir for saying this but I think that is just how you are behaving—as a judge

Dr Emerson: You must of course say what you think, but I am the responsible person here.

Dr Scott: I know that Sir.

The value of this dialogue is not in whether or not you agree with it, but in encouraging you to consider your own views on the subject and test these against others.

Books written by patients about their own experiences of illness are of course uniquely useful and illustrate some of the real difficulties that they face. For example, Anne Dennison's book, *An uncertain journey*, describes her feelings and experiences of living with cancer. Henrik Ibsen's play *'Enemy of the people'* shows very clearly some of the problems related to public health when an individual doctor wishes to take action, which is against the wish of the community, to improve health. The play offers a remarkable insight into dealing with public health, and the naivety of the doctor becomes clear.

Looking at problems surrounding issues of death and dying, a little book of poems by Douglas Dunn entitled *Elegies* illustrates the issues well, and records his feelings while his wife was dying:

Thirteen steps and the thirteenth of March
She sat up on her pillows, receiving guests.
I brought them tea or sherry like a butler,
Up and down the thirteen steps from my pantry.
I was running out of vases.

More than one visitor came down, and said,
"Her room's so cheerful. She isn't afraid".
Even the cyclamen and lilies were listening,
Their trusty tributes holding off the real.

Doorbells, shopping, laundry, post and callers,
And twenty-six steps up the stairs
From door to bed, two times thirteen's
Unlucky numeral in my high house.

And visitors, three, four, five times a day;
My wept exhaustions over plates and cups
Drained my self-pity in these days of grief
Before the grief. Flowers, and no vases left.

Tea, sherry, biscuits, cake, and a whisky for the weak. . . .
She fought death with an understated mischief—
"I suppose I'll have to make an effort"—
Turning down painkillers for lucidity.

Some sat downstairs with a hankie
Nursing a little cry before going up to her
They came back with their fears of dying amended.
"Her room's so cheerful. She isn't afraid."

A further poem by another author, which illustrates the problems of being in hospital, is entitled 'Marooned'. It tells the story of a woman and her fellow patients who were stranded in a hospital dayroom, unable to move, without support:

They set off in convoy to the dayroom
They were settled in the round
The TV was blaring loudly
And drowned out every sound

Relative peace was established at last
Relaxation, satiety, a dream

For some moments at least things were better
Than sometimes they often might seem

But then crisis occurred foreseen
But not quite anticipated
No sticks or zimmers available
They were suddenly isolated

There was a babble of female voices
Some silent, some loud, some slurred
All eyes showed fear and fright
The TV blared unperturbed

No one could move, marooned,
The place was just like a tomb
Locked and sealed, cut off
Transformed from a hospital room

For a time, the length doesn't matter
They sat slumped alone in the chairs
No one seemed to be worried
Who was concerned with their cares?

Marooned, they sat, marooned,
Others quite unaware
Marooned at the heart of a hospital
Marooned in a sea of care

And if you wish to look at life in the 1990s, as opposed to historical novels, *Trainspotting* by Irvine Welsh will show the whole panoply of emotions, concerns, and sexual attitudes faced by those involved in the drug scene, HIV infection, and alcohol. Roddy Doyle's book *'The woman who walked into doors'* is a remarkable study of domestic violence.

There has been an emphasis on books which illustrate human problems or disease issues. This of course is not the complete story. Literature as a whole is relevant and enlightening. Indeed, the comments from students indicate that books and plays which are not of an overt ethical or medical nature are equally valuable, if not more so, in helping to understand values and moral issues.

2. Art and music in the hospital

What then about art in hospital? This can be viewed in two ways. First, the use of paintings, murals, tiles, and sculptures within hospitals to enliven surroundings and to create an atmosphere of healing rather than illness. The importance of design, of attention to detail cannot be underestimated. Similarly, with the buildings themselves, architecture can be a vital part of the therapeutic experience. So many hospital buildings seem to give little attention to use of space, colour, and texture. Secondly, there is the use of art to express emotion and illustrate concern, in turn, encouraging debate and discussion. Indeed, one of the key themes related to the humanities and medicine is the importance of engaging people in discussion in order to consider, think through, and understand more fully their own views and those of others. The use of art as therapy both in adults and children may be a valuable part of rehabilitation and self-awareness. Creative writing for patients and professionals can be part of this.

Music in hospital is important both in terms of therapy, and also for allowing people to relax, to think, and to have their own feelings explored and expressed more clearly.

3. The arts and the public

Arts in the community are of course also very important, and some remarkable schemes have been developed. In the Craigmiller Housing Estate on the outskirts of Edinburgh, over the last 20 years or so, there has been a music festival encouraging and developing individuals, and producing remarkably creative results. This has been well documented in a book by Helen Crummy, *Let the people sing*. In Withymoor Village Surgery in the West Midlands, there has been an attempt to explore, once again, both the general role of the arts and music within the community and their role in healing. In Bromley by Bow in London, a church has been transformed into a centre for creative arts involving the community and using the enormous range of skills which are available. Music in Hospitals is a charitable organization which supports a range of musical events for patients.

4. The humanities and clinical practice

Many of the arguments in this chapter are addressed at people's ability to talk, converse, and understand their own feelings, and to be able to communicate these to others. This issue of communication is crucial. Studying the humanities allows us to see how creative people can think through an individual situation, and gives us insights into human emotions and feelings which can help us to understand the importance of our own feelings and of communicating these with others.

In relation to clinical practice, the humanities encourage an holistic view of care. We should think beyond treatment to care itself, and consider issues such as emotion, compassion, and the ability to listen. Within this, and central to it, is the importance of patient input into the whole process. Their involvement, participation, and commitment to improving health and health care, as partners, is obviously essential.

Issues surrounding the humanities in clinical practice and medical education have been debated for many years, and continue to be. The debate is perhaps typified by that in the early years of the century between Flexner, someone who felt that the scientific base of medicine was crucial, and Osler, who considered that a broader education which included issues beyond medicine was also important[5]. The issues they raised remain alive today. In any organization, particularly a learning organization like the National Health Service, the ability to think beyond the need for trained individuals to solve immediate problems, to having those with the skills, ability, and expertise to respond to new problems and challenges. This needs an educated person.

5. The implications for managers

Managers too have to make important decisions which involve not only judgement and dealing with uncertainty, but also creativity and thought beyond their own particular experiences. For that reason, and as a teaching tool, the use of literature, art, and music are particularly important. For non-executive directors, particularly those coming from outside the health care system, the experience of thinking through some of the books and poems which have been illustrated in this chapter may give them greater insight into some of the difficulties faced by patients and professional staff.

In conclusion, it can be reckoned that a broader educational experience and an appreciation of the humanities allows professional staff to link their own values to wider values, to consider a greater range of emotions, and to become attuned with feelings. Books, plays, and poems are very important ways to improve learning and are useful teaching tools in this respect. They also, however provide great relaxation for those concerned. For the future it is necessary, that the education of doctors, nurses, and managers should encompass issues beyond the technical aspects of dealing with particular problems to encourage a more rounded and educated person. With the full involvement of the patient, the result will be to improve the quality of care.

References

1. Calman, K. C., Downie, R. S., Duthie, M., and Sweeney, B. (1988). Literature and medicine: a short course for medical students. *Med. Ed*, **22**, 265–9.
2. Calman, K. C. and Downie, R. S. (1996). Why arts courses for medical curricula? *Lancet*, **347**, 1499–50.
3. Downie, R. S. (1994). *The healing arts. An illustrated Oxford anthology.* Oxford University Press.
4. Calman, K. C. (1997). Literature in the education of the doctor. *Lancet*, **350**, 1622–3.
5. Tauber, A. I. (1992). The two faces of medical education: Flexner and Osler re-visited. *Journal of the Royal Society of Medicine*, **85**, 598–602.

7

The medical detective

One of the principles set out at the start of this book was a need to have effective mechanisms for the monitoring and surveillance of health and the outcomes of health care. There is more to it than that, however. It includes the need for curiosity and questioning, and for a culture which constantly seeks to find out more and to explain the reasons for disease and its consequences.

1. The role of intelligence in health and health care

Doctors have many different roles: clinician; manager of health care and resources; and, importantly, medical detective, looking for and interpreting clues to diagnose disease and illness. This is relevant both to the individual patient and to the community as a whole, and is driven by the natural curiosity of doctors. This curiosity, together with the need to improve health and health care and to act on the intelligence, ensures that wherever possible problems are identified and prevented.

This chapter therefore asks a series of questions. How do you look for clues? Why did it happen? Could it have been predicted? Can you explain it? What can we do now? And what are the consequences? The relevance of identifying such problems can be illustrated with two brief quotations:

When trouble is sensed well in advance it can be easily remedied . . . so it is in politics. Political discords can be healed quickly if they are seen well in advance. *Machiavelli.*

Epidemics resemble great warning signs on which the true statesman is able to read that the evolution of his nation has been disturbed to a point which even a careless policy is no longer allowed to overlook. *Virchow, 1848.*

An examination of the detective in fiction can illustrate key characteristics of some of the issues. Consider, for example, Sherlock Holmes—a character based on a real-life Edinburgh doctor, Joseph Bell, who had an uncanny ability to make a diagnosis as soon as the patient walked into the consulting room. Sherlock Holmes reveals the same talent:

'And the murderer?'
'Is a tall man, left-handed, limps with the right leg, wears thick soled shooting boots, and a grey cloak, smokes Indian cigars, and carries a blunt penknife in his pocket.' (From *The adventures of Sherlock Holmes).*

Other detectives in fiction such as Morse, Hercule Poirot, Smiley, and Brother Cadfael all display different methods of solving problems and identifying clues. In most instances they carry out a great amount of routine detective work and it is within this that unusual clues appear. And it is precisely the same in health and health care—hard work and shoe leather are required.

What then is intelligence?

Intelligence can be seen as evaluated information and acts as an early warning system for problems which lie ahead. Its purpose is to assist in decision making, in planning, and in prediction. In population terms these comments are relatively easy to understand. At the clinical end, with the individual patient, the intelligence system of the doctor is continually looking for clues about the patient, their illness, and the possible response to treatment. Taking it a little further it also looks for clues as to why the illness was caused in the first place and whether or not there are features which are out of the ordinary. Thus seeking intelligence has both diagnostic and prognostic functions; diagnostic in the sense that it allows the pattern of illness or disease to be recognized from the clues available, and prognostic in that it allows decisions to be made about the future course of action and possible progress of disease.

Intelligence however is rarely complete and this is the case not only for the detective, but also for the clinician and epidemiologist. There is a need to work with degrees of uncertainty, and always, a requirement for judgement. It is the ability to take one step beyond the information available, based on the intelligence gathered, which can often result in an earlier diagnosis or the prediction of a clinical problem. Looking for clues therefore is about uncovering unusual facts based on a great amount of routine data gathering.

Turning information into intelligence

In trying to systematize information and convert it into properly evaluated intelligence, there are perhaps three issues which need to be looked at. The first is to identify people who may have special skills, and are at the leading end of clinical or public health practice. These are individuals to watch, to learn from, and to listen to. The second is to identify particular clinical issues—HIV infection, cigarette smoking, breast cancer, or whatever—and to be sure that you are able to keep up to date with what is happening, what is changing, and, wherever possible, to be ahead of the game. The third is to look at interesting or unusual patterns of disease or of clinical findings; these are often the ways by which new problems are uncovered. These three elements combined with searching the literature and keeping in touch with individuals through well-developed networks, mimic the ways in which intelligence services around the world look for clues in the vast amount of information which is collected about people, problems, and patterns.

Much of this of course requires an understanding of the natural history of disease. The influenza which lasts longer than it should, the abdominal pain that does not settle within a few days, the unusual neurological symptom which is not explicable—all alert the clinician to the fact that something is changing and is not quite right. The well-known saying that 'chance favours the prepared mind' is one which can be illustrated many times in clinical and public health practice. For a sporting analogy, the story is told of the famous golfer who had just had an excellent round. It was commented that he must be very lucky, to which his response was 'The more I practice, the luckier I get'.

Sources of intelligence

If then we are to concentrate on people, problems, and patterns, what are the sources of intelligence that we can use? Clearly contacts and networks are exceptionally important; knowing who to get in touch with and how to ask them for information is central to this, requiring a knowledge of the databases available and the ability to use them effectively. The doctor needs to establish such networks and to develop contacts which will continually bring to him, or her, or other health professionals, information about changes in disease patterns or management. It is for this reason that developments in information technology such as the internet are now so much part of clinical practice.

2. Some examples of intelligence

It is not difficult to find examples of how individual clinicians or public health doctors have identified issues which have been important in improving the health of the population. One such example concerns Sir George Beatson, a surgeon in Glasgow, who while working on a farm in the 1890s noted that the removal of the ovaries of sheep changed their pattern of lactation. This observation was made before hormones were discovered but led him to make the suggestion that removal of the ovaries from a patient with breast cancer might result in its regression. He carried out the experiment and showed that hormones had a significant effect on the development of breast cancer. A second important example would be that of identifying the relationship between cigarette smoking and lung cancer—one of the most important observations in clinical practice this century. Moving to drug therapy, one particular example relates to an incident in Bari Harbour during the last war, when troops were exposed to an unacceptably high level of nitrogen mustard. This resulted in the fall of the white blood cell count in the soldiers. A very astute pharmacologist recognized this and suggested therefore that the drug might be helpful in the treatment of leukaemia, which has a very high level of abnormal white cells. This was the beginning of a very successful way of treating the disease. New technologies and discoveries in medicine need constant evaluation and assessment. The Research and Development Directorate in the National Health Service—the Health Technology Assessment Programme—fulfils that function and is increasingly used to evaluate new diagnostic and therapeutic techniques.

3. The consequences of the intelligence function

The prediction of health

Receiving intelligence of a change in health or health care is one thing. What it means, and what can be done about it is another. There are several consequences which can be identified, the most important of which is the ability to predict health both for the individual and for the community. This is a very important concept and relates to earlier discussions on the purpose of health and the importance of quality of life. As there may be implications on the quality of life of that individual, there is clearly an ethical dimension to predicting health, which will be discussed later. For almost all of the determinants of health and those factors which influence health care it is possible to set up an intelligence system which will begin to predict relevant issues.

It is not difficult to find examples of the prediction of health which are well established. Age, for example, predicts health, as does the sex of the individual, whether or not they smoke, and social class. Looking at one particular issue, maternal fetal interactions, it is possible to identify the fact that the health of the baby is likely to be affected by radiation, smoking, the nutritional status of the mother, viruses, and drugs which may cross the placental barrier. All of these factors (and perhaps in the future, even more will be identified) can affect the health of the baby, both in the long term and the short term. This is one of the most exciting and interesting areas of clinical practice. Taking another example, infant mortality, it is possible to single out those areas of the country where the rate is higher, and a wide variety of illnesses can be predicted by the social class of the parents. Infant mortality rates are also clearly related to the weight of the baby at birth; the weight itself gives a clear prediction of possible survival.

Communication of intelligence

The second consequence of intelligence gathering, and therefore the prediction of health, is how best to communicate this to the public or to individual patients. As has been discussed elsewhere communication is perhaps the key to this whole issue. The ability to communicate risks is not an easy thing to do and must be done with great care, taking account of the need to build up trust with the patient and the population. This trust is central to delivering important messages about risks to individual or population health. This is discussed more fully in Chapter 4.

Managing incidents

Once intelligence shows that an incident may occur, for example, the outbreak of infection or of an environmental problem, then it is necessary to take rapid action. This requires teamwork and the involvement generally of a wide range of professionals, the public, and the media, together with communication of the actions to be taken. Over the last few years the ability to communicate throughout the health service, and in particular with doctors, has improved. The use of electronic mechanisms has facilitated such communication, providing information to allow those concerned with the identification or management of a particular disease to be brought rapidly up to date.

Ethical issues

The fourth consequence of intelligence and the prediction of health relates to the ethical issues which may be raised. As has been previously discussed, the role of ethics is to clarify thinking, assist in analysis and decision making, and to help in managing uncertainty. Basic human values are often in conflict and the rights of the individual and the needs of the population may not always be at one. The intelligence, or the clues which may be uncovered, can relate to one or many different segments of the population, and the consequences may therefore be quite varied. This is particularly highlighted when the subject of genetics and health is raised. It is increasingly possible to identify single- or mulitple-gene abnormalities in patients, and to relate these to particular conditions. The ability to do this, and thus to predict health with much greater accuracy, does raise some very fundamental ethical issues. Many of these are of course not new, but are highlighted by such new information. They include the need for confidentiality, the implications and consequences of screening patients, employment problems such as disclosure to the employer of health information, the exploitation of such information, and the importance of consent and insurance issues. All of these are well-recognized and current problems.

The concept of a 'genetically disadvantaged' person is possible. These are people who may appear normal but are known to have a gene for a particular disease or illness. Just as individuals who have physical handicap may be discriminated against, so such genetically disadvantaged people may have the same problem. In addition, it is important to note that while the knowledge of a disease may be personal to an individual and their own doctor, if that disease is hereditary then it does have relevance to the offspring of the patient. This does mean that the consequences of passing on such information to others, and giving them an 'equal weight' in the knowledge of the diagnosis, needs to be considered. This 'principle of equal weight' is of great importance, in view of the potentially devastating consequences to the affected individual (including those relating to insurance) should genetic testing be done.

Another factor relates to the interaction between the environment and the genetic characteristics of the individual. It is possible to foresee a situation in which an individual has a gene which makes them more or less susceptible to such things as food, smoking, or alcohol. If this is the case, what responsibility does the individual have to modify their behaviour on the basis of such important genetic information? These are just some of the ethical issues raised as a consequence of the intelligence function.

4. The role of patients and the public

Throughout this book it has been stressed that patients and the public need to be involved in issues of health and health care. So it is with the gathering and analysis of intelligence. The role of the individual or the patient cannot be overemphasized, nor can their need to be involved in such issues. They have a positive role as collectors of information and intelligence, and they have a unique experience of the problems.

5. Some conclusions

From this review it can be seen that the intelligence function is a basic one for the doctor or other health care professional. However, the consequences of identifying clues need to be considered carefully and include predicting health, communicating risks, managing incidents and taking action, and dealing with the ethical problems which are thereby uncovered. Much of this, of course, depends on attention to detail and the ability of the doctor to see unusual patterns or a natural history which has something out of the ordinary.

Two further quotations from Arthur Conan Doyle's detective, Sherlock Holmes, summarize this perfectly: 'You know my method. It is founded on the observation of trifles' and 'To a great mind nothing is little'. (From *The adventures of Sherlock Holmes*.)

Being a medical detective is great fun. It is an exciting part of clinical and public health practice. It offers the chance not only to be 'ahead of the game' but also to solve practical problems for the patient and for the public at large.

8

The science and art of public health

'You should never have your best trousers on when you turn out to fight for freedom and truth.'* Ibsen, *The enemy of the people

1. The science of public health

Introduction

Public health may be defined as 'the science and art of preventing disease, prolonging life, and promoting health through the organized efforts of society'. It is therefore about people and how the health of the people can be improved. It was Francis Bacon who said 'Human knowledge and power coincide because ignorance of a cause hinders the production of the effect', showing how closely related knowledge is to the power to change. In a splendid book, *Pioneers of health*, by M.E.M. Walker, 12 of the great pioneers of public health, whose names are carved around the building of the London School of Hygiene and Tropical Medicine, are identified. All are important because of the scientific advances they made. In considering previous Chief Medical Officers in the Department of Health, four of the first five were Fellows of the Royal Society—indicating once again the value of the science and research base. The first conclusion therefore is that public health has always had, and always should have, a strong science base.

Some basic issues

Though many people have tried to set out the importance of measurement in science, it was perhaps Lord Kelvin who put it most succinctly. He said 'I often say that when you can measure what you are speaking about, and express it in numbers, you know something about it'. And, as an extension of this, there was the implication therefore, that if you could not measure something it was difficult to describe. Peter Medawar, who has again written a great deal on science, says 'The word science itself is used as a general name for, on the one hand the procedures of science . . . and on the other hand the substantive body of knowledge that is the outcome of this endeavour'. Also that 'Science is organised knowledge . . . and this organisation goes deeper, than the conventional ologies.' From these statements it can be seen that science may be viewed as a method, a knowledge base, and a discipline.

One issue which may need developing further, therefore, is a theoretical base for health and healing. There are a number of possible models available which allow for the prediction of health or the effectiveness of healing on outcomes of health care. These models provide the basis for further work and for the evaluation of interventions; some are described in Chapter 1 of this book. They can also be used to define the science base of public health. Public health is an amalgamation of a series of 'ologies'. It does not draw on one single science but on epidemiology, molecular biology, clinical practice, sociology, education, politics, and management science. Hence the importance of team work and of using a wide range of skills to improve health. One way of looking at this is to view the population as a public health laboratory—a population which can be studied, and whose health can be understood. The knowledge base which can be derived from such studies provides a way of seeing how health can be modified for the better. The establishment of the determinants of health—which include environment, lifestyle, biological factors, social and economic issues, and health services—are a step in the right direction, but more is needed. In particular, better tools and measuring instruments to ensure the clearer definition of issues and outcomes. In addition to this, the knowledge base must have an intelligence function which identifies, at the earliest possible moment, changes in health (see Chapter 7). The intelligence function and the research base are clearly linked. In carrying out such studies there are also ethical implications, and these too must be considered in improving health.

The second conclusion therefore is that although the scientific basis is well established in public health, there needs to be improvement in the methodologies used, and in their range.

Where are we now?

It is not difficult to consider a wide range of interventions in public health and to ask a fairly straightforward question as to the evidence of their effectiveness. Several issues immediately come to mind: the value of exercise; the role of nutrition; the importance of risk assessment; and factors involved in behavioural change, such as cigarette smoking. In each of these the problem can be clearly identified and the question formulated, but there is still a lack of data which links the epidemiological information of the risk factor with the change which needs to occur if health is to be improved.

In academic terms public health also needs to be developed further. There is a continuing necessity for a forum to discuss research issues and new developments, and a clear need to ensure integration between the academic departments of public health and the public health service function. The link between service and academia is one of the great strengths of British medicine, and it must be promoted further. In addition, links with other 'non-medical' scientific disciplines are clearly crucial if the specialty is to develop more. We need to give very careful thought to the infrastructure for science and public health, and the need for proper funding.

Future issues

Looking back, there have been very considerable achievements in medicine and public health practice. It is an interesting exercise first, to identify what the key issues have been and, secondly, to look ahead and try to single out those areas which will be important over the next 20 years. This topic is developed further in Chapter 13. Issues of considerable interest for the future include genetics, molecular biology, screening, behavioural science, and socio-economic issues. One exciting area for development is forging the link between social and economic factors, such as deprivation and poverty, and the clinical effects of morbidity and mortality. Molecular biology is one interesting component of such a link. For example, the research on prenatal events makes it clear that social and environmental factors can have long-term consequences. These consequences must also have a mechanism, such as effects on the neurological, endocrine, metabolic, or immunological systems. Molecular epidemiology is a new science and one which may reap many benefits. In the future perhaps we will be discussing more frequently the molecular basis of public health, a prospect raised later in this chapter.

A further conclusion, therefore, is that we need to retain the science base, improve the training, and identify the major issues ahead.

Some conclusions

Looking ahead, two anecdotes help to set the scene. The first is the story of the appointment of the first Medical Officer of Health in Edinburgh, Sir Henry Littlejohn. He was appointed in 1864 after a tenement in the High Street in Edinburgh collapsed killing a number of people. In the midst of the rubble a little boy was heard to say 'Heave a wa' lads I'm no deid yet'. The reconstructed building has the face of the little boy and that motto carved above the door. The moral here is that public health is seeing a renaissance. With a strong science base it can take off and ensure improvements in health. The second anecdote concerns Sir William Tennant Gairdner. He was the first Medical Officer of Health in Glasgow and subsequently became Professor of Medicine. In an address to the British Medical Association in 1883 he said that 'the limitation of sanitary functions to men, not engaged in medical practice, and of medicine and surgery to person who are thereby exempt from all preventative duty will not be without serious disadvantages. It will tend to split the medicine into two sections, perhaps into two more or less hostile camps'. This again contains a fascinating lesson: it is important that public health becomes integrated fully into the main academic streams and that its links with clinical medicine are strengthened.

This section began with a quotation from Francis Bacon and it concludes with another: 'Man who is the servant and interpreter of nature, can act and understand no further than he has, either in operation or in contemplation, observed of the method and order of nature.' This emphasizes the importance of observation and scientific study in improving health, and the public health doctor has a responsibility (as a servant and interpreter of nature) to be part of the process.

While the scientific basis of public health is clearly of importance, it is also vital that such findings are put into practice. The practical implications of public health are an art and require special skills in themselves. These skills need emphasizing and developing and include both management and political skills and skills in the communication of ideas and complex public health issues. This leads directly into a consideration of the art of public health.

2. The art of public health

In the previous section the scientific basis of public health was discussed, together with some related implications for the practice of public health based on the use of available evidence. In this section the art of public health will be reviewed which, in essence, is about how the science can be put into action. The objective of both is the same, however—to improve health, health care, and quality of life of the individual and the community. The art of public health therefore is about 'making it happen', setting the agenda and following it through. It is the craft of translating a public health issue into improved health. The outcome is the important end point, and the means of getting there may vary from issue to issue. As in most things change comes about through people, not paper.

The art is to effect change, based on the best available scientific evidence. Knowledge itself is neutral and inert; it is what is done on the basis of the evidence which is important. To change health is not a simple or an easy process—if it were then we would all be much healthier now. The potential is there if it could only be realized. This section sets out some of the issues related to public health which need to be considered if health is to be improved, and draws some conclusions which might assist in the process.

1. Has the problem been clearly defined? There may be a tendency to assume that simply by stating the problem, answers and action will follow. This is not necessarily the case, as not infrequently, the wrong questions are asked. Over the past few years there have been a number of such instances with the result that the follow-through to action has been delayed or missed. The science and knowledge base remains crucial and the facts cannot and should not, be changed to suit a particular agenda. The conclusion therefore is that the problem and the question should be clearly defined.

2. What is the strength of the evidence? While the importance of the evidence has been emphasized it is also relevant to consider the strength of the evidence. There is little point in constructing a major health campaign or initiative on the basis of insubstantial evidence. The information required for effective action concerns not only the science and the quantification of the effect on health if the policy is to be successful, but the value for money of the proposed changes. For example, cigarette smoking is probably the major health hazard in this country. Almost anything which would reduce the take up of smoking, or result in smoking cessation by more than 1 per cent, would be a significant step forward. Conversely, if a substantial financial input into some other health issue results in only a small health gain, then it might need to be questioned.

The requirement to set out in a very clear way the health gain which might be expected by changing, for example, the environment, behaviour, or lifestyle, should be self-evident if those who make the decisions are to be convinced. Health gain must also be related to the cost of the change in human resources, facilities, and finances.

3. The timing of the initiative This may be one of the most importance features of the art of public health. So often the issue is right but the time is wrong. In these circumstances it is important to recognize the difficulties and to avoid pushing too hard in case outright rejection occurs. A strategic retreat is sometimes the best course of action.

4. The importance of having several initiatives Because of the difficulty of getting the timing right it is necessary, at any one time, to have a number of topics which might be pursued. These may not arise in any logical order, so it is important to have all the issues relating to each topic ready, to activate at any time. Concentrating only on one issue can limit effectiveness in the long term if opportunities for change appear and they have not been prepared for.

5. From incident to innovation In some instances a public health incident can provide the opportunity to develop an initiative which, under other circumstances, would have a much lower priority. The art of public health is to be ready to exploit such incidents for the benefit of the community. Just as in clinical practice where the doctor has two roles—to treat the illness and to help the patient benefit from it—so the public health practitioner has the same responsibilities; to deal with the problem, and to look ahead to population benefits.

6. What are the implications for change? Managing and effecting change is never easy and can be difficult to carry out. For this reason it is necessary to consider in some detail the consequences of the proposed changes on the public, patients, professionals, and resources. Unless these are considered at the planning stage, potential problems will not be addressed.

7. Who are the key players? Early on in the process of change it is essential to identify those who will ultimately make the decisions. These include politicians, local government officials, and the media—and not just those concerned with health. People skills are central to the art of public health; influencing, advocating, convincing, informing, supporting, and assisting are all part of this. Key players will vary with the issue, which may be national or local.

8. Presenting proposals for change A great deal of time and energy needs to be put into getting the problem on the agenda, though it should be remembered that the submission of a well worked-up proposal may not be enough. Time needs to be spent on informal discussions and meetings, and on gaining ownership. Equally if there is no support for the proposal at an early stage it is probably best to regroup, revise the proposal, and consider the timing afresh, rather than push ahead and end up with an outright rejection. This may seem to be a protracted approach, but it is important to remember that it is winning the war which is the long-term objective—the first skirmish is not important.

9. How will the action be followed through? Getting the idea right, amassing the evidence, considering the implications for change, and influencing the key people will not be sufficient unless there is an effective plan and an implementation strategy. This will include an assessment of the resources required. The grand idea alone is not sufficient, it needs a practical programme for making it happen.

Some examples of change

Over the last 50 to 100 years health in Britain has changed dramatically. In most instances—lifespan, infant and maternal mortality, reduction in infectious disease—the change has been an improvement. There has been a major shift from infectious disease to those conditions more associated with lifestyle. While socio-economic conditions have improved considerably, they remain a significant influence on health. Some problems remain however (cigarette smoking would be one of these) and it is interesting to ask why certain initiatives have been successful and others have not, and to see if lessons can be learned which will improve health. The skills required for the art and craft of changing health may thus be defined more clearly in this way.

The following might be considered to be some of the important changes which have occurred to improve the public health:

- immunization programmes for childhood diseases
- clean water and safe food; sewage disposal
- health and safety regulations
- Clean Air Acts and air quality regulations; lead-free petrol
- the use of seat belts and drink driving laws
- safer homes and the reduction of accidents
- the introduction of a national health service
- the provision of maternal and child health services
- medical advances such as antibiotics and blood transfusion
- public education and awareness about health
- improvement in the general level of education.

These might be classified in four ways: first, the role of Government in the regulation of matters which will affect health; secondly, the provision of a health service available to all; thirdly, improvements in medical practice, education, and research; and fourthly, the role of all those who supply information and education to the public (this would include the voluntary sector, the media, and the Government).

Medical research is clearly a professional responsibility (though funding is often from government sources); others have a strong sense of government involvement. The value of those doctors and scientists working in the government service, and their role in influencing policy development, cannot be overemphasized.

Why do people change?

If one of the significant components of the art of public health is to be able to influence the people who make decisions, what can be done to direct the process? Several factors are relevant including:

- the presentation of new information or evidence
- the influence of colleagues and personal friends
- pressure from the media or the public
- the occurrence of opportunities arising from incidents
- the cost-benefit ratio moving in favour of change

People can sometimes change rapidly, but more often it takes time, and this may be necessary if the decision maker is to have ownership of the outcome. Change, for an individual, often depends on the environment in which it is to occur. Indeed, the environment may be one of the most important determinants. A person may wish to eat more fruit and vegetables, but if these are not readily available this may be difficult. A person may wish to take more exercise, but if the culture is such as to make him or her feel unusual, the change may not occur. The perception of the issue may be incorrect and time is needed for new information or ideas to be assimilated. Patient and quiet persistence are often rewarded. In most instances the credibility of those providing the information and the new initiative is critical. Hence the importance to the art of public health of relationships and networks. Going out on a limb rarely helps. Again, the role of those in government service—both in research and service positions—in promoting public health issues at a national level is emphasized. The partnership between those in government and those at the sharp end is crucial.

The role of civil service doctors

For almost 150 years there have been full-time doctors working in the service of the Government. At present they work not only in the Department of health and its agencies—the Medicines Control Agency and the Medical Devices Agency—but also in the Home Office; prison service; the Departments of Transport, Defence, Social Security, and Education; the Health and Safety Executive; and the Office of National Statistics. They bring a very wide range of expertise to the posts and, through their networks, intelligence of changing patterns of health and health care. They have an important function of assessing evidence and presenting it to ministers. Their strength lies in their close working links with policy makers and ministers, which allow them to influence policy formulation. They provide an independent and impartial view. Distinguished medical civil servants in the past can claim to have had an important place in improving the health of the nation. Those who want to improve health could do no better than join the medical civil service. The job of the Chief Medical Officer is the best public health job in the country.

Some principles which emerge

From the discussion so far some general principles about the art of public health can be discerned. These are not new and nor are they specific to public health, as the biblical analogies used below make clear:

1. 'Cast thy bread upon the waters . . .' (Ecclesiasticies, 11). Put your investment in several places because you never know what kind of bad luck you are going to have in this world. Every public health doctor needs to have a range of issues to hand, ready for any opportunity which might present itself.
2. 'To everything there is a season, and a time for every purpose under the heaven.' (Ecclesiasticies, 3). Timing may be everything and the public health professional must be prepared for all eventualities.

3. The need to spend time on having the right seed (the evidence) and on cultivating the soil (the decision makers). (Luke, 8). Investment of time and energy in this process will reap rewards.
4. Foundations need to be secure, and a good idea is not sufficient. The concept needs to be built on solid rock, and be able to withstand criticism and debate. (Matthew, 7).
5. 'If one of you is planning to build a tower he sits down first and works out what it will cost . . . to see if he can finish the job.' (Luke, 4). A plan is required which considers the implications for resources and implementation—without this the idea will come to nothing.

In practical terms the process needs to be set out in a coherent way, and the following are some of the personal lessons learned over the years.

Stage 1
This is concerned with generating and clarifying the idea. It involves testing the water by meeting and discussing with key people the issues involved. At this stage a paper may be unhelpful, but there should be some indication of the likely support for the idea. A decision then needs to be made as to whether or not to progress with the issue.

Stage 2
Pen is put to paper and a very short document is produced to give direction to debate. Once again a round of informal discussions and meetings are held as the structure of the paper becomes clearer and the views of others are taken on board. Ownership is crucial. The timing and support are again reviewed. If favourable, the process moves to the next stage.

Stage 3
This consists of getting the topic on the agenda of the right group, with a properly worked-up paper which has already been agreed by some, if not all, members of the group. The timing may still not be right or the evidence convincing. Even at this stage a return to Stage 1 should be contemplated.

Stage 4
This consists in the follow-through and evaluation of the project. It will again involve meeting people and maintaining the momentum.

The hitchhiker's guide to public health

In searching for an analogy to illustrate the way in which the art of public health is put into practice, the vision of the hitchhiker appeared attractive. It gives the image of an explorer, or discoverer; someone resourceful who can adapt to meet needs; someone who knows where he or she is going and is prepared to use a range of methods to get there. The steps taken by the hitchhiker set out some of the issues already discussed, but in a rather different way:

1. The hitchhiker needs a map of the whole area, and to be clear about where he or she wants to go. Detailed plans of some parts of the map will also be required, together with links to on related regions or countries.
2. The hitchhiker must be able to take opportunities. He may want to go to Brighton but the first lift he gets is to Crewe. He could wait and hope that the right bus or car will come along, or he could get started right away.
3. During the expedition different modes of transport may become available, and each may have their uses, advantages, and disadvantages.
4. The hitchhiker needs to have a haversack containing both tools and resources, food, and a change of clothes in case there is bad weather ahead.
5. A list of things to do when reaching the next destination is essential. Turning up and not knowing what to do will just waste time, and an opportunity may be lost. Adequate forward planning is essential.
6. Finally, at the end of the journey, he or she needs to sit down and reflect on the lessons learnt on the trip and begin planning the next one.

The art of public health is long, and the journey continuous, moving from one topic to another, using a wide range of skills and experience. In some instances new ways will have to be found to change health, but that is the challenge. According to an Aboriginal saying, 'There are no paths, paths are made by walking'. The excitement of being in public health is in making new paths and in discovering new ways to improve health, a comment which leads into the next area for discussion, that of research.

3. The potential of research affecting the socio-economic approach to prevention

A practical public health problem

Many examples could have been chosen to illustrate the role of research in an area of public health. This particular topic is not only important in itself, but highlights some of the difficulties and challenges.

Introduction

There is considerable evidence for the relationship between social and economic factors and health.

The question however is why? how is it possible to explain the relationship, and can mechanisms and models be identified which describe the way in which the health consequences can be understood? The first part of this section sets out some of the background issues and the context and covers the purpose of health, health promotion and prevention, the relationship between socio-economic factors and health, and quality of life. The subsequent section on research builds on this groundwork. For a more detailed discussion of poverty see Chapter 2.

The promotion of health and the prevention of illness

The title of the section assumes that it is clear that the objective is prevention of ill health. But this is not sufficient and the aim can be interpreted more widely to cover:

- preventing ill health
- reducing disability
- improving quality of life.

Social and economic factors also have a bearing on access to, and use of, health and social services. For this reason another category needs to be included:

- improving outcomes of health care.

The research implications of each of these will be developed further in subsequent sections of the book.

The relationship between socio-economic factors and health

The relationship between society and the economy is a complex one, though they are clearly interdependent. Society makes choices on how to use its resources; the economy and its growth influences society; and both are related to the health of the population and of the individual. The major factors which determine this relationship between society, the economy, and health are the values within the particular society, which may vary with time and with different cultures. However, this needs to be examined at a research level if it is to be understood and explained. Thus, an explicit statement of the values underpinning society and how it uses its wealth is important if the relationship is to be comprehended.

Economics

Economics is generally defined as how people allocate scarce resources amongst competing uses to maximize their satisfaction. Gavin Mooney puts it this way: 'Economics is about choice; it is about opportunity cost; it is about maximising the benefit to society from the resources available'. The science of economics thus has two important characteristics; namely choice and satisfaction. It is both about the common good (for the community or the population—macroeconomics) and individual quality of life (microeconomics). It covers public wealth and private income. It is an exciting discipline, and one cannot agree with Thomas Carlyle who said that 'Economics is the dismal science'.

The role of economics in national terms, therefore, covers:

- resource allocation and choices
- use of the workforce; employment
- growth-output per head
- maximizing satisfaction.

Economic factors

Under this heading could be grouped all the factors relevant to the production, distribution, and consumption of wealth that have an impact on health. Which economic factors do have a vital influence on health in any particular society is difficult territory, but those factors commonly quoted include:

- the rate of economic growth
- the level of distribution of national income
- consumption patterns
- the relative prices of healthy or unhealthy goods and services
- the incentives and disincentives of tax policies.

The importance of some of these factors may be contentious, while for others it is proven. For example, tobacco prices and hence tobacco taxation is one of the most important determinants of preventing smoking that can be directly influenced by government.

Social factors

A wide variety of issues can be grouped under this heading, all of which are related in one way or another to health. Indeed almost all factors which determine health can be covered under this heading, including genetic factors, which in some instances may be related to family or cultural aspects of social life. Relevant factors include:

- family, friends, and social networks; social structure
- work/occupation as well as employment status
- home and environment
- lifestyle
- ethnic factors
- isolation and transport
- urban and rural issues
- level of education attainment.

The research issues surrounding these factors present difficult challenges. In addition it should not be assumed that these factors always operate in one direction; that is, the lower the social class (however defined), the greater the implication of poor health. In some instances, for example in malignant melanoma, the opposite is true.

Quality of life

This is at the heart of the relationship between social and economic factors and health. People have choices to make, albeit sometimes limited, the end point of which is satisfaction. These personal choices are contingent upon social and economic factors. Health, or the health consequences of adopting a particular lifestyle, may not be the dominant factor. Other issues may be perceived to be more important. Short-term and long-term consequences are also relevant for each individual.

All of this relates to the fact that quality of life (satisfaction) may be expressed not only in terms of physical illness, but in psychological, emotional, and spiritual ways, each of which may be considered important. Thus quality of life is a key issue, and one based on personal values (see Chapter 10).

The way ahead

How can we view the way ahead? This section, as has already been stated, is not about action to deal with social and economic factors, but research. There is no challenge to the fact that relationships exist, and that they constitute major areas of health and social policy, at the heart of which is social justice. A great deal of evidence is already available. The Our Healthier Nation strategy has one important and unique feature which supports this—the Cabinet Sub-Committee, representing 11 government departments, collaborates and co-ordinates the gathering of such evidence. We have an opportunity to build on this part of the strategy.

4. Research

Interests for the research worker in this field are huge, but only four main areas can be considered here:

(1) documentation and descriptions of the relationships between social and economic factors of health;
(3) development of research tools;
(3) evaluation of interventions;
(4) explanation of relationships.

1. Documenting the relationships

An initial question which must be asked is whether or not we need to do more? Do we not already have sufficient descriptive epidemiology? The answer is probably no, although we do need to be clearer about the questions, otherwise we will simply be reinventing wheels. Some of the issues which might be looked at further include:

a. Income and health, and their relationship with time and other variables. The relative effects of different incomes need more clarification.
b. Natural history studies on the implications of occupational status, immigration, and cultural factors. For example, the differences in the levels of schizophrenia in the community require more scrutiny.
c. Housing and health. This has long been the object of study. However several issues remain to be described in detail including the consequences and relative health effects of homelessness, and of some putative factors,

such as dampness. This would give some quantitative data on the investment required to improve health, and what the gain would be.

d. Further studies on factors operating prenatally, antenatally, or in early life. This might include social status and nutrition.
e. Violence, including the important issues of accidents, injuries, and suicide. This represents a major problem in society. Yet its origins and characteristics need further study.
f. The role of women. Women remain the main carers in society and a most important source of health information. As such, they, together with children, constitute a key group.
g. Changes in social structure need to be documented. Single-parent families are frequently at greater risk than most. Greater specificity is required in asking the questions.
h. Studies on specific groups such as school children. This is a particularly interesting group as social class seems to be much less relevant in adolescence.
i. Educational attainment. This is a major determinant of health. Yet the data is less well known than it might be.
j. Access to health care. We need to know more about why some groups use health care more than others, but more importantly, about the health consequences of such variables. Quantitative data on mortality, disability, and quality of life are all relevant.
k. Behavioural epidemiology. It would be helpful to have more information on further behavioural characteristics of populations and groups. For example, to say that teenage girls continue to smoke, does not explain why, and more detailed work is required. There is a need to generate hypotheses and to test them.

2. Development of research tools and methodology

While much is available, we clearly require more sophisticated tools to analyze issues such as quality of life and with which to relate environmental factors and health risks. We also need to ensure that we have adequate databases and national survey material (for example, the National Food Survey, Health in England Survey) with which to work. Finally, the necessity to understand motivation and behaviour must be self-evident. We have some instruments to study this but we could do with more.

3. *Evaluation of interventions*

Each year we make substantial investments in health and in health promotion—smoking cessation, dietary advice, health and safety issues, and so on. It is essential that such initiatives are evaluated and their effectiveness identified. Such evaluation needs to include a social and economic perspective, to isolate those interventions which are particularly effective. We should also recognize in planning interventions for a whole population that selective uptake might actually increase the inequalities. For example, if smoking reduction interventions are more effective in the higher social classes, then the differences between the groups may widen. Of particular interest are ethnic minority groups, whose response to improving access to health care, for example, may require specific resources and methodologies.

The investment of resources—including skills, time, facilities, and funding—into health needs careful monitoring if the full potential is to be realized.

4. *Explaining the relationships*

So far the discussion has concentrated on issues of a descriptive nature. For many factors the final common pathway is clear, for example, smoking in lung cancer, risk factors in occupational health. But two issues remain. First, why do the behavioural patterns start in the first place, and second, how is it possible to explain those aspects, such as stress, which appear to have no obvious mechanisms? Research, therefore, is urgently needed to explain the variations in health. Why, for example, is there a higher mortality in lower grades of civil servants than in higher ones? How is it possible to explain this, or develop a model which connects work with mortality? Is it possible to consider a molecular mechanism which links stress with subsequent mortality? Is it possible to relate a psychological problem to the haematological changes which occur before a myocardial infarction?

Three broad areas of research thus need to be considered: behavioural mechanisms; neurobiological implications; and the possible biochemical or immunological consequences of social and economic factors. Each of them require further research much of which will be at a basic level and may come from unrelated disciplines dealing with different problems—and the development of methods and instruments. Hence the need to ensure a critical mass of expertise to enable collaboration and co-ordination to take place. Essentially, the required research can be summarized as:

a. *Behavioural studies* It is clear that social and economic factors influence behaviour, but much more work is required to define the mechanisms, and to look at group effects and peer pressures. In particular the research might be directed towards why certain behaviours are taken up, and the social interactions which influence them. Some of these questions are not new, but the results of such research need to be made more widely available and used to underpin educational programmes. Hypotheses have to be generated and tested.

b. *Behaviour and neurobiology* Our understanding of how the brain works has advanced significantly in the last few years. The need to integrate this very basic work with behaviour studies, and social and economic factors, is exciting.

c. *Molecular mechanisms* There is considerable research in other fields which shows that stress results in significant changes in endocrine status, biochemical measurements, and the immune response. Some of these changes are likely to have health consequences and yet few studies have been done to link social and economic variables with such changes. Stressful events, for example, a surgical operation or an illness, show such changes and in the 1930s Sir David Cuthbertson outlined the concept of 'ebb and flow' after injury. In these studies he showed that after stress there was an inevitable flow from the body of protein and other metabolic products. After a period of time, which related to the severity of the injury, these flowed back and the patient recovered. This model was an acute one, and it would be of interest to follow this up with a mechanism involving chronic stress, and to test the ebb of metabolic products and psychological coping mechanisms. The implications would be that the 'flow' which precedes recovery might be delayed or absent. The psychological insight into using the concept of 'ebb and flow' should also be relevant.

Is it therefore possible to postulate an hypothesis which explains variations in health in relation to social factors to account for those aspects which are as yet unknown? It might be presented as psychological factors such as stress and loss of control cause metabolic changes which lead to changes in health, mediated via:

- endocrine changes
- acute phase reactants
- interleukins and interferons
- melanotonin
- immunological changes.

Each of these, individually or collectively, can change the possibility of an event which might have a health consequence occurring, and there is evidence that they do so. We urgently need population studies which will examine these issues and develop the techniques of molecular and cellular epidemiology.

This section has outlined some of the research issues involved in looking at social and economic factors and health. They are fascinating and fundamental, and at the heart of improving health. What is missing is not the large epidemiological study but a multidisciplinary team of epidemiologists, biochemists, neurobiologists, behavioural scientists, and immunologists to work together on this topic.

5. Some final thoughts

This chapter has set out a range of issues concerning the science and art of public health. It is an exciting time to work in this field; the potential is enormous. In the recent past, medicine and science have concentrated mainly on two of the three daughters of Aesculapius—Panacea and Iaso (the healers). In future we should perhaps pay more attention to their sister Hygeia. If we do, then the future looks bright.

6. A postscript on hygiene

Words, like clothes, are fashionable and have significances and meanings which change with time. So it is with hygiene. It has gone in and out of fashion, but perhaps its time has come again. Hygiene, as a concept, was particularly prevalent in the late nineteenth century, with developments in sanitation and sewers. Hygiene, in the broadest sense, is the science of health. If ever there was a need for such a science it is now. We need a strong evidence base, and the development of models which will show new ways of dealing with public health problems. Research is fundamental to this.

Hygiene is also used in a much more restricted way to mean issues of personal cleanliness, and the proper preparation and storage of food. Once again the need to relearn the old lessons are clear. Skills in cooking are much less obvious than they were, and there is an assumption that modern medicine will be able to deal with any minor issues of food poisoning. This is not always the case, and such infections are not always minor and not always treatable. Simple rules exist which, if followed, will help to reduce the incidence of infection and ensure that protection of the public health is maintained. They include:

1. Wash hands thoroughly before preparing food, after going to the toilet, or handling pets.
2. Prepare and store all uncooked food separately from cooked food—keep raw meat or fish at the bottom of your fridge.
3. Keep the coldest part of your fridge below 5 °C. Get a fridge thermometer. Keep eggs in the fridge.
4. Keep your kitchen clean. Wash worktops, chopping boards, and utensils between handling food which is to be cooked and food which is not.
5. Defrost frozen meats and poultry fully (in the fridge or microwave) before cooking, unless the cooking instructions state otherwise.
6. Cook food thoroughly, following the instructions on the pack. If you reheat food, make sure it is piping hot.
7. Undercooked meat—particularly burgers, sausages, and poultry—can cause illness. Take extra care to cook them thoroughly until the juice has run clear and no pink bits remain. Do not eat food containing uncooked eggs.
8. Keep hot food hot and cold food cold—don't leave them standing around. Take chilled and frozen food home quickly, putting them in your fridge or freezer at once.
9. Check 'use by' dates. Use food only within the recommended period.
10. Keep pets away from food, dishes, and worktops.

Further reading

Walker, M.E.M. (1930). *Pioneers of health*. Oliver and Boyd.

9

International aspects of health

'No man is an Island entire unto himself' **John Donne**

1. Introduction

International aspects of health affect us all, and the brief consideration of the issues here can do no more than outline some of the major topics. For further information the publications of the World Health Organisation (WHO), the World Bank, the United Nations Childrens Fund (UNICEF), and other organizations should be consulted. This chapter has three main themes. First, that international aspects of health have general implications which are relevant to this country. Second, that the main issues in health across the world are remarkably similar, though associated with different patterns of disease. And third, to emphasize the relationship between economic growth and health, and the intersectoral nature of health improvement. The information used in this chapter comes from the 1995 World Health Report from the WHO in Geneva. The European data is from WHO's Copenhagen office. Further helpful information comes from the 1993 World Development Report on Health Status from the World Bank.

2. The impact of international aspects of health

In a developed country like the United Kingdom international aspects of health have several implications. The first relates to communicable disease which, with the ease of transport, is ever more freely transmitted to populations across the globe. Movement of populations for business, leisure, and migration is occurring on a scale as never before. The great epidemics of the past (plague, cholera, influenza) and of the present (AIDS, tuberculosis, malaria) show just how vulnerable the world is to such infections. The introduction of quarantine in Italy and France in the fourteenth century was one of the earliest attempts to control such infections. The second implication relates to environmental issues, the most recent and serious of which was the radioactive release in Chernobyl. Environmental problems regularly cross international boundaries, as the effects of acid rain and global warming make clear. The need to ensure that there is an environmental impact assessment of economic growth has been set out in a series of programmes, as part of 'Agenda 21'—the UN initiative on the environment and 'sustainable developments' for the future. The third factor acknowledges that the richer countries put considerable resources into improving health in the developing world, and they need to be sure that in doing so, they obtain value for money from the investment. The fourth factor concerns migration and immigration. As already stated, considerable population movements occur across the world, generally from those areas which are poorer, or in regions of conflict, to the richer parts of the world. Movement of people, and with them, changing patterns of disease, provide a living laboratory in which to investigate the aetiology of certain illnesses. For example, the cancer incidence in some populations changes considerably following migration, and this gives clues as to causation.

These four factors represent a clear justification for all countries to have an interest in international aspects of health.

3. Some current health problems

Levels of health, measured in almost any way, vary considerably from country to country. The collection of accurate statistics and their analysis is the responsibility of the WHO, the World Bank, and other international organizations. They show the extent of the problems:

1. 30–40 million adults with HIV infection by the year 2000 (cumulative total); 10 million cases of AIDS (cumulative total).
2. 3 million deaths from tuberculosis each year—5 per cent of global deaths; estimated 2 billion carriers.
3. 300–500 million people with mental illness, including neurosis and psychosis.
4. 2 million deaths from malaria in 1993.
5. 350 million chronic carriers of Hepatitis B; 1 million deaths in 1993.
6. 100 million people with diabetes by the year 2000.

In the UK the infant mortality figures for 1996 were 6.0 per 1000 live births. In some other countries, figures for the same year of 140 to 160 deaths per 1000 live births are recorded. Life expectancy at birth varies from around 40 years in the poorest countries to over 80 in the richest. These are huge variations and the economic cost of this burden of disease, ill health, and disability, is considerable. In the same year the USA spent 2800 dollars per person on health, compared with 2–40 dollars in the poorest countries.

At the same time as countries develop, health and lifespan improve, and the problems of an ageing population become clearer. (The rise in the elderly population is occurring worldwide.) The factors which influence the variations or inequalities in health between countries are well known. In the next section, health in Europe will be considered to illustrate these issues in more detail, and there will be a general discussion of those factors which affect health inequalities.

4. Health in Europe

Over the last few years a considerable amount of data has been collected on health in Europe, the most recent being the report by the WHO European Regional Office in Copenhagen in 1994. The information used here comes from that Report. The European Region ranges from Portugal to Russia, from Iceland to Turkey, and includes the countries of central and eastern Europe (CCEE) and the newly independent states (NIS) such as Kazakistan, Belarus, and the Baltic states. The number of countries in the European Region of the WHO has risen from 31 to 50 in the last few years.

Certain general factors are relevant. In 1992, no less than eight countries were affected by war, with the consequences of conflict such as violent death, disruption of the infrastructure, and migrations of several million people. In countries of eastern Europe in particular, an economic recession has had a major impact on health statistics, as will be described shortly. The migration of large numbers of the population has been associated with poverty, homelessness, and poor living conditions. Violence has been obvious in many countries. What have been the implications of these changes on the health of the people of Europe?

Life expectancy in the countries of the European Union (EU) continues to rise and is, on average, around 72 years for males. This is in contrast to a number of countries in the NIS where life expectancy has actually fallen. While this is a crude indicator of health it demonstrates how rapidly changes in circumstances—social, economic, and environmental—can have an effect. Infant mortality in Europe ranges from 5–10 per 1000 live births in most nordic and western European countries, to over 40 in some central Asian republics. Generally the figures show an improvement, but in some CCEE and NIS countries there has been a slight increase. Maternal mortality is similarly distributed, and is again declining overall.

There are considerable variations in cardiovascular mortality across the European Region of the WHO. What is particularly disturbing is that between 1985 and 1992, while many countries showed a decline in mortality (the UK by 5 deaths per 100 000), others showed considerable increases. The lessons of prevention will need to be learned all over again in the CCEE and NIS. In a similar way, age-standardized death rates from cancer in the 0–64 age group are decreasing in the EU and nordic countries, but increasing in the CCEE and NIS. Higher smoking rates and alcohol consumption explain some of these differences.

In terms of communicable disease the overall results indicate that they remain a major health problem. Polio, diphtheria, and cholera have all seen a resurgence. Immunization rates are generally high but in some of the NIS protection against, for example diphtheria, is inadequate. The health service infrastructure is such in some countries that it is difficult to implement vaccination programmes. Tuberculosis is increasing, partly due to migration of very large numbers of people. By August 1994, there had been a cumulative total of 116 000 cases of AIDS reported in the Region. Encouragingly the annual incidence shows signs of slowing down, thanks to huge preventive efforts over the last 10 years.

Women's health is of special interest. Maternal mortality is high where abortion remains the principal method of contraception. There is particular concern about the cigarette smoking rates in women, and the mortality in women from lung cancer continues to rise. Finally, in this snapshot of figures, the number of elderly people in the Region continues to rise and they are a distinctively vulnerable group. Mental health problems also are a cause for concern in all countries of the world.

The picture therefore is a mixture of good news and bad, with substantial lessons to be learned. The main issues from the preceding two sections will now be discussed.

5. Factors influencing international variations in the levels of health

This brief review allows some general conclusions to be drawn:

1. **The importance of the economy**

Poverty and the rate of economic growth are clearly linked to health. There is very considerable international data which supports the link between the two, and they are related in a cyclical way: poverty decreases health which produces a poor workforce which decreases economic productivity; economic growth produces wealth which improves health and provides a better workforce. It is not possible to separate the impact of the economic state of a country from poverty and the level of health.

2. **The intersectoral nature of the potential for health**
There is an increasing need to integrate health measures with housing, social services, and environmental concerns. For most improvements in health, the requirements are not for better hospitals or specialist facilities, but for clean water, safe housing, and the production of safe food.

3. **Educational level**
The level of education of the population is closely related to health status. This is particularly the case for women. In Kenya, for example, for women who have had more than seven years' schooling, there is a 50 per cent reduction in the mortality of their children compared to those who have not been educated. Such a clear demonstration emphasizes the special role of education and its priority in improving health.

4. **The role of women**
All reports stress the role and rights of women, and their essential place in society. Women make decisions about food, health, and lifestyle and are therefore the most important agents for change. Violence against women, and the restriction of their role are particular problems.

5. **Violence and war**
Occurring across the globe, war places human life at grave risk and disrupts the provision of services, including food and vaccination, from which it may take years to recover. Violence generally is increasing in some societies, perhaps as a result of lifestyle changes such as the abuse of drugs. Domestic violence is of particular concern. In both cases it extracts a toll on the health of the nation, and shatters the health infrastructure. The role of international health agencies and humanitarian organizations is especially important during times of conflict.

6. **Health services**
The level of provision of health services is of considerable importance particularly in relation to the balance between hospital and primary care, the use of resources to develop effective interventions, and the ability to deliver public health measures. The infrastructural organization and management are both important.

For most health care systems, primary care is the most important feature. It was enshrined as a basic principle by the WHO in the declaration of Alma Ata in 1978 (see Chapter 2). The conflict in the use of resources in developing countries between primary care and the acute hospital sector may be of a different magnitude to that in the developed countries, but the issues are the same. How do you ensure the most effective use of limited resources to benefit the greatest number of the population? The draining away of resources to specialist facilities instead of towards primary care is thus especially relevant.

For developing countries a number of interventions are known to be both effective and affordable. These include immunization, information on family planning and infant and maternal health, reductions in the use of alcohol and tobacco, improvements to environmental conditions such as air and water, the treatment of tuberculosis with short courses of chemotherapy, and the underpinning of an appropriate diet with vitamins, iodine, and iron. The development by the WHO of the essential drug list is very much part of this, and all of this can be delivered within the primary care setting.

It can be argued that hospital services are needed, even in the poorest countries. However, in this situation it is necessary to ensure that the treatments are effective and the outcomes give value for money. The professional challenge in developing countries, as in this country, is to measure and evaluate outcomes of care. For this reason good management of the resources available is essential, and one of the requirements in developing countries is to ensure that such management skills are available. In many countries of the world a reassessment of the structure and organization of health services is proceeding, to make them more effective and to achieve value for money. Many different models are being tried and it is necessary to ensure that the lessons learned in one country are shared with others. One of the values of international health organizations is that they can be used to facilitate the sharing of such information.

6. Health for all

The slogan 'Health for all by the year 2000' was first adopted by the WHO in 1978, and has served two main purposes. The first was in setting a general aspirational objective, a kind of philosophy which has been very useful in assisting governments in developing health policies. The second was to associate this objective with a target date, and to also set a series of quantifiable objectives or targets. The European Region of WHO, for example, in 1984 set 38 targets for the Region as a whole, covering topics from equity to ethics. Some, in areas such as heart disease and smoking, were very quantitative. Many countries in the Region now have national policies which have similar objectives covering similar topics. For other regions of the world the use of the Health for All strategy has been of great benefit, although it is clear that the overall objective will not be reached by the year 2000. This does nothing to negate the concept, but will require a greater focusing of effort on to those topics which will achieve the greatest health gain for the population as a whole. We have much to learn from how other countries have tackled their health problems. This is discussed in more detail in Chapter 2.

7. Ethical issues in international health

In general the ethical principles outlined in Chapter 5, of justice, autonomy, utility, non-malevolence, and beneficence, are relevant in international health issues. However, there are some specific topics which cross boundaries and which serve to illustrate the complexities of global health problems:

1. **Equity**
This is perhaps the most important of the ethical issues. In the interests of justice, equity is a principle which must be sustained. The information given earlier in this chapter shows just how variable the levels of health are between countries.
2. **War and violence**
The ethical and moral dimensions to war and violence have been discussed throughout the centuries. The 'just' war may or may not have an ethical foundation, but the impact of war on health is clear. Torture is one aspect of this.
3. **Women's issues**
In some countries of the world women have few rights and are treated as second-class citizens. Gender-based violence is common. Genital mutilation is still practised in some places. As has been discussed several times in this book, women are crucial to the health of the population. Unless they are treated equitably, an important consequence of justice, then health will suffer.
4. **Advertising**
As the advertising of tobacco becomes progressively more difficult in some countries, so the manufacturers have turned their attention to the developing world, and the huge markets which are opening up there. As these countries become more affluent, so the consumption of such products increase, with consequent long-term adverse health effects.
5. **The ethical promotion of pharmaceuticals**
In countries with limited resources the need for effective drugs to be supplied as cheaply as possible is essential, and the use of expensive alternatives avoided. Heavy promotional campaigns can divert resources, hence the importance of the WHO Essential Drug Project in offering economic drug supply.
6. **Reproductive health issues**
One of the major problems in the world at present is over-

population. Methods of contraception are readily and cheaply available, and have very few adverse effects. Yet abortion continues to be used for contraceptive purposes in some countries, with its associated health consequences. In some countries religious views oppose the use of contraception in any form. This therefore takes the arguments for and against contraception from an individual perspective to a national one. This is a good example of how the value system and beliefs of a nation or culture can affect the health of the population. Unplanned parenthood and multiple pregnancies can have many health and social consequences, and are closely related to the role of women in society.

7. **Investment in health**

As in this country, how money is invested in health can be of considerable importance. Donor agencies—humanitarian organizations—put much money and skills into developing countries. In doing so it is essential that priorities are set to achieve the maximum health benefit. Some of the issues raised earlier in this chapter about effective interventions are relevant. The balance between the allocation to primary health care or hospital care would be an example of this. It is important that with limited resources available the right choices are made, but who is to make these choices? The country itself or the donor agencies? The arguments here are entirely analogous to those discussed in Chapter 10 on resource allocation.

8. **Breast milk substitute**

All health authorities are clear about the value of breast feeding for the mother and the baby. However considerable pressure might be brought to bear on mothers in developing countries to use breast milk substitutes. Not only would this be more expensive, but the health benefits of breast feeding would be lost. International action was required to deal with this issue and the World Health Assembly resolved that there was to be no free or subsidized milk substitute, which would affect breast feeding practice.

9. **Racial and religious differences**

Issues of race and religion feature strongly in terms of conflict and discrimination. The moral principle of justice argues that all should be treated equally and fairly, and that there should be both equality of opportunity and of access to health services. Repression and discrimination against minority groups can have profound health consequences and result in major variations in health outcomes. In ethical terms these variations are not defensible if the principle of justice is to be upheld.

8. Partnerships in health

There are now a very wide range of organizations dealing with international health issues. The WHO has six regional offices, each of which links closely with other organizations. For example in Europe, the WHO European Office has close links with the European Union, the Council of Europe, the Red Cross and other humanitarian agencies, the World Bank and other major donors, individual countries, and other international funding agencies. All of this needs to be co-ordinated if duplication of effort and a waste of resources can be avoided. Each of the agencies has a particular advantage and it is essential that they work harmoniously together. As stated before in this book, ownership of improving health is required, and it means changing 'health for all' into 'health by all' to demonstrate the need for real involvement by all concerned.

9. Summary

The issues described briefly in this chapter have highlighted a number of general principles and illustrated the basic problems which are of relevance in any country which wishes to see the health of its citizens improved. They include the importance of social and economic issues, the intersectoral nature of action, the role of women, the level of education of the population, the organization of health services, and the way resources are allocated.

The action required in each will be discussed later in the book.

Further reading

WHO, Geneva. (1995). *World health reports, 1995, 1996, 1997.*
WHO Copenhagen (1994). *Health in Europe.*
World Bank. (1993). *World development report.*

10

Health care

1. What is health care?

Health care is that part of influencing or improving health which requires advice, a service (including early diagnosis and prevention), treatment, or care to be given to an individual or community. This service may be provided by the individual (self-care), by family or friends, by a voluntary organization, or by professional staff. The purpose of this process is to improve health, relieve symptoms, or supply comfort. This is well summed up in the phrase: 'Guérir quelquefois, soulager souvent, consoler toujours.'—(To cure sometimes, to relieve often, and to care always.)

Health care is thus concerned not only with curing disease, but with providing care and compassion. In assessing the value of the care provided (generally by measuring the outcome of the process) it is not sufficient therefore to be concerned only with the measurement of end points such as death or the incidence of side-effects of treatment—the whole approach to care, including quality of life, needs to be considered. This can be very difficult to assess. However, if such an holistic approach is not adopted the patient will be seen only as the 'appendicitis in bed three', rather than as a person with a complex series of needs. As will be discussed later, the outcome of care, as set by the patient and the team at the start of the process, is of increasing importance as a way of allocating resources and monitoring the quality of the care provided. This, however, is not easy and requires the patient to be a partner in the process.

Who is it that provides health care? For most illnesses, care is provided by non-professionals, including the patient himself, and is delivered in the context of the home and the family. Only a small proportion of the care required is referred to the primary care team, and an even smaller amount to the hospital and specialist sector. This is a phenomenon which occurs in all cultures. It is for this reason that the home, and women in particular, are so important. It is also the reason why members of the public require information about health and health care in order that they can make appropriate decisions about the need for further help. As medicine advances, and expectations rise, so the public may make more and more use of professional time. The balance between what can be offered for self-limiting illness and the need for specialist input is constantly shifting. Greater public information on its own may increase the use of professionals, rather than decrease it, if it is not accompanied by practical educational programmes. The increasing role of the media in alerting the public to health issues is a positive way forward, but can lead to an increasing demand for health care. Awareness of new treatments or diagnostic techniques can lead to greater use of services, and stimulate demand. Still it must be remembered that it is the public who deal with most illnesses, and it is the professionals who are there to serve the needs of the population as a whole.

While this chapter will be concerned mainly with the ways in which a high quality of health care can be delivered, it should be noted that there are very strong links to education, patient involvement, research, and ethical issues—all of which are covered in more detail elsewhere in this book.

2. Quality of life

Increasingly quality of life is being discussed in relation to health care. It is no longer sufficient to measure only length of life or remission, the quality of life of the patient needs to be considered. That said, quality of life is difficult to measure or even to define. Clearly quality of life can only be described and measured in individual terms, and depends on present lifestyle, past experience, hopes for the future, dreams, and ambitions. Quality of life must include all areas of life and experience and take into account the impact of illness and treatment. A good quality of life might be said to be present when the hopes of an individual are matched and fulfilled by experience. The opposite can also be said to be true—a poor quality of life occurs when hopes do not meet with experience.

Quality of life changes with time, and under normal circumstances can vary considerably. The priorities and goals of an individual must be realistic and would therefore be expected to change with time and to be modified by age and experience. To improve quality of life therefore it is necessary to try to narrow the gap between hopes and aspirations, and what actually happens. The aim is to help people to reach the goals they have set for themselves. A 'good' quality of life is usually expressed in terms of satisfaction, contentment, happiness, fulfilment, and the ability to cope. From this definition, certain implications follow:

1. It can only be assessed and described by the individual.
2. It must take into account many aspects of life.
3. It must be related to individual goals and aspirations.
4. The goals must be realistic.
5. Improvement is related to the ability to identify and achieve these goals.
6. Illness and treatment may well modify these goals.
7. Action may be required to narrow the potential gap. This may be taken by the patient alone, or with the help of others.
8. The gap between expectation and reality may be the driving force for some individuals.
9. As each goal is achieved new ones are identified, opening the gap again. It is a constantly changing picture.

Quality of life, therefore, measures the difference, at a particular moment, between the hopes and expectations of the individual and that individual's present experiences.

Quality of life has many dimensions covering all life areas including home and garden, work, hobbies, financial issues, body image, diet, mobility, ambitions, spiritual issues, and concepts of the future. The identification of problems and priorities makes it possible to develop realistic goals and to use these to assess progress and measure the change in the 'gap'. Thus can the interventions be evaluated. This model is discussed further in Chapter 1. Oliver Wendell Holmes puts the issues of dimensions of quality of life more eloquently in *The professor at the breakfast table*:

> The longer I live the more I am satisfied by two things. First that the truest lives are those that are cut rose diamond fashion with many facets. Second that society in one way or another is always trying to grind us down to a single flat surface.

Several new methods are now available to measure quality of life, some based on the wide range of dimensions just listed. They are essentially problem based, identifying areas of life—such as pain, a financial problem, a failure to cope with a difficult issue—that require change or support. In all however, it is the difference between hopes and reality which are relevant. Dr Johnson put it well:

> I know not anything more pleasant, or more instructive than to compare experience with expectation or to register from time to time the difference between idea and reality.

In practical terms it is the relationship between length of life and quality of life which needs to be clarified, and for this it is necessary to return to the earlier discussion on the purpose of health (Chapter 1). It will be recalled that the purpose of health was to contribute to quality of life, and that health was a means, not an end. If this is accepted, then an extension of life without at the same time increasing or maintaining its quality would not be considered valuable. Immediately a series of ethical problems arise between choices and objectives of treatment. Because of the uncertainty of outcome in many instances it will not be possible to face this with the clarity which might be wished. Hence the importance of patient involvement and choice.

The overall objective is to reduce the period of ill health, disability, morbidity, or side-effects, while increasing lifespan. Thus to 'compress morbidity' until the end of life would be the ideal, the patient having only a short period of disability or symptoms. The implementation of the Our Healthier Nation strategy will only be relevant to the population as a whole if this objective is achieved.

3. Quality of care

***'I think there is such a thing as quality, but as soon as you try to define it it goes haywire. You can't do it.' Zen and the art of motor cycle maintenance*, R. Pirsig**

Over the last few decades we have seen remarkable advances in health care. Diseases which were untreatable can now be cured. New drugs, diagnostic procedures, and surgical operations have changed the lives of millions of people. And advances will continue, allowing people to live longer and with a better quality of life. The care provided through the National Health Service is of a very high standard, and in general practice and in hospitals around the country, patients receive up-to-date and high-quality care. But how can we be sure of this? How can this statement about care be justified? How can the quality of care be assured in all hospitals and from all doctors, nurses, physiotherapists, dieticians, health visitors, and so on? This section sets out how this is being done and how it might be improved. But first some introductory remarks.

Attempting a definition

Quality is not easy to define, as was discussed earlier in this chapter. The first thing to remember, however, is that quality is everyone's business, and all members of the care team need to be involved. This means setting and meeting standards, and continually improving and updating them. The following definition tries to encapsulate some of the more important issues involved:

'Quality is a concept which describes in both quantitative and qualitative terms the level of care or services provided. Quality as a concept therefore has two components. The first is quantitative and measurable, the second is qualitative and associated with value judgements. It is a relative and not an absolute concept.'

It is not simply therefore an analysis of activity. In describing the quality of a particular service it should always be compared to some other similar activity, previous measurements, or value judgements. It also implies consistency over a period of time in the delivery of a service or care.

Quality can be related to the achievements of specific aims, objectives, standards, or targets. These standards however should not be seen as fixed, as they can always be improved. In describing the quality of a service all those involved need to be considered—doctors, nurses, receptionists, porters, and managers, as well as the patient and the family. The morale of a hospital department has a direct effect on the quality of care.

From this definition it can be seen that quality is a relative concept, not an absolute one. The quality of care provided is therefore related to the individual's own past experience and to the performance and expectation of others, including patients, the public, and politicians. To improve quality means being able to do better than you are doing now. The starting point of all quality initiatives is therefore an assessment of where you are and where you want to go; the measurement of quality is change and the rate of a change. Some changes will be readily measured, others will be more difficult and require judgements about the kind of service provided.

Areas for assessment

Above all quality is about values. If you really believe that something is valuable or worthwhile (communication, education, relief of pain, and so on), then it is likely that you will wish to take special care with it. For that reason it is the values given top priority by the organization, or clinical team, which are most important. If the manager says that communicating with relatives and patients is essential, and actually does it, it will set standards for others to follow. Leadership is very important.

If we were to be able to assess the quality of care provided by the doctor, how might it be done? As quality is multidimensional, several different areas would need to be reviewed, and while the following example is related to doctors, other professional groups could be discussed in a similar way. Areas for review might include:

(1) technical skill and competence, for example, the ability to perform certain procedures, prescribe drugs, and make appropriate clinical assessments;
(2) standards of professional behaviour, including ethical and moral issues;
(3) attitudes, including communication skills and appropriate responses to patients and families;
(4) managerial functions, including leadership—all clinicians have a responsibility for managing resources and there is also a quality dimension to this;
(5) teaching, research and development, and clinical audit.

For each of these inter-related functions it is possible to begin to define standards and to monitor the outcome. Equal weight need not be given to each of the components since, to some extent, the speciality and grade of the doctor will have a bearing. The medical component is of course only one part of the process. In a similar way it is possible to list a series of categories which might be used to measure the quality of a clinical department:

(1) a clinical records system in place which documents relevant information and is regularly checked for quality;
(2) identification of the common procedures or illnesses seen by the unit, for example, a list of the 5–10 conditions most frequently dealt with;
(3) guidelines or standards set for each of these conditions or procedures, including information for discharge and follow-up;

(4) clinical audit procedures in place to monitor quality and the standards set in the guidelines;
(5) documentation of all new procedures introduced with evidence of effectiveness and an evaluation of the outcome;
(6) evidence of involvement of the patient or public in the work of the unit, for example, in the production of the guidelines, information leaflets, patient participation groups, and so on;
(7) staff appraisal systems in place to give feedback on the quality of care provided;
(8) documentation of educational programmes and opportunities available to all staff—a crucial part of quality assurance;
(9) teamwork in evidence, utilizing the skills of all staff;
(10) the management of resources including time, skills, facilities, and finance, as evidenced by an awareness of staff of the consequences of mismanagement.

Setting and measuring standards

This then raises the question as to who should measure the quality of a doctor or a clinical unit? If the list related to doctors is considered first, several issues arise. First, doctors should have a responsibility themselves for measuring the quality of the care they provide. This can be done through audit and peer review, and is an integral part of clinical practice. This applies to all other professional groups. In general, the first issue on the list, technical skill and competence, is probably best assessed by other doctors, but all of the others would benefit from an assessment from other professional staff or managers. The public also have a role in this process in ensuring that the standards of care which are set out by the professions are being met.

In a similar way the list of quality issues related to a clinical unit which are proposed should be assessed by the team itself, but there is a clear role for those outside the unit, including managers and the public, to be involved. As is discussed in Chapter 12, the professions, because of the high standards of care they provide, have no need to be concerned about public scrutiny. They can welcome it as a method of assuring the public of the quality of care given. The possibility of accrediting a clinical service by a special team might even be considered.

Finally in this justification of the high standards of care provided in this country, who should set the standards and how are they to be controlled? In general it is the professions themselves who set standards. In medicine, the General Medical Council (GMC) and professional bodies such as the Medical Royal Colleges are the ones who through professional mechanisms and self-regulating functions, set and monitor standards. Within the GMC there is a specific group of non-medical people who have a responsibility for overseeing this process. In addition, at the level of the hospital or general practice, managers have a responsibility to ensure that the care provided is of a high quality and to offer the public reassurance and involvement.

An important philosophical question is whether or not the standards set should be 'minimum' or 'gold' standards. As quality is always a relative term, it is perhaps unwise to set 'gold' standards as they are likely to change and be improved. Setting minimum standards is also not entirely satisfactory as it assumes a very low base from which to start. In general, some kind of level which equates to 'good' clinical practice will be chosen and regularly monitored, updated, and revised. As with most educational processes, it must begin at the level the team are at, and build from there.

Control and monitoring mechanisms

What are the tools available to assist with the process of change? There are a number of them, and all have a place. To echo the words of Mark Twain, 'If your only tool is a hammer, all your problems will be nails'. Some of these mechanisms have already been mentioned, and others will be discussed in more detail in subsequent sections. They include setting explicit standards of care, developing guidelines for good clinical practice, and having in place systems of clinical audit which will monitor standards. There are a number of 'sticks' available to assist with this including the GMC procedures for poor performance, the sanctions of the Royal Colleges for teaching and training posts, and employers responsibilities for ensuring that clinical staff whose practice is poor are identified. Educational programmes for retraining are available for those for whom it would be appropriate. There are in fact, for the profession as a whole, very few 'carrots' other than professional pride in good performance. Perhaps, however, the key is to create a culture of quality and excellence as the norm and part of good professional practice. This would set a social context in which certain standards of behaviour and professionalism are built into the educational and training programmes. This requires leadership and high-quality practice at the top of professional groups.

4. Outcomes and effectiveness

It seems self-evident that it would be a good thing to measure the outcome of the process of health care. There are many ways of assessing the process by measuring activity (beds used, number of patients seen, waiting times, and so on) but these give no estimate of the outcome or of its quality. The previous discussion has shown that measuring quality is not straightforward, and setting standards and developing guidelines not a simple matter. As outcomes are the end point of the process they are therefore the key to assessing quality. Some examples will help to illustrate the issues:

1. **Asthma**

This is an illness which is increasingly common and measuring the outcome is therefore important. The use of mortality figures is not very helpful as fortunately the mortality rate is low. It might be possible to estimate the frequency of admission, but this will also reflect referral patterns. The type and frequency of use of medication might be another method of measurement. For patients a good outcome is likely to be related to less time off work or school, and being able to sleep at night. Neither of these last two components of information is collected locally or nationally.

2. **Palliative care**

The outcome, in most instances, is death, which is readily measured. The real issue however is about measuring the quality of life before death occurs and, as discussed elsewhere, this can be a very difficult thing to do.

3. **The results of surgical operations**

In some ways these outcomes are easier to measure and might include mortality at times after the operation; the incidence of postoperative complications or side-effects, short-term or long-term; time to rehabilitation; and patient satisfaction with the process.

From these three examples several general principles emerge. First, there are often several different outcomes which can be measured, and in some instances the data for these is not routinely collected. Secondly, there may be differences between the outcome as perceived by the patient and by the professional—the old saying 'the operation was successful but the patient died' springs to mind. Thirdly, the time at which the outcomes is measured—soon after the procedure or some time later—may be crucial. Finally, the difficulty in measuring outcomes needs to be highlighted.

What then are the general factors which affect outcome? Just as there are a number of factors which influence health so there are several factors which affect the outcome of health care. These include:

1. The health status of the individual. This can sometimes be forgotten. The health of the person at the start of the illness can affect his or her ability to respond to treatment. For example, a person who is overweight before a surgical operation is more likely to have subsequent complications. Pre-existing disease such as diabetes or tuberculosis can also affect the outcome. If the population as a whole, for

example, is malnourished or has coexisting infectious disease, then the impact of treatment may be affected.

2. The disease, its natural history, the stage at diagnosis, and the prognosis. This is often the major determinant of the outcome of care in terms of survival and response to treatment. For example, a patient with influenza will generally get better after a few days no matter what treatment is used, though it is possible to alleviate symptoms. For patients with lung cancer, the type of disease and how far it has spread is the major determinant of outcome. It is essential that the public recognizes that until new treatments are available, this will be the most important factor in influencing the outcome of this disease.

3. The treatment available. This is clearly important. For some diseases the treatment is very effective, for example, the use of antibiotics for a bacterial infection. In others it is less so. Even antibiotics may not be effective in all cases, and side-effects can occur.

4. The skills of those providing the treatment and care. This is the educational and training dimension of outcomes and may be the limiting factor in providing high-quality care. It is, of course, not just about the ability to provide a technical procedure, but also to give comfort and care, and to communicate effectively.

5. Facilities and resources available. If the necessary machine or diagnostic equipment is not available then the options to improve outcomes become limited. This includes the range of skills offered, together with the resources to provide the care required. It is a complex issue and will be discussed in more detail later.

This section demonstrates the necessity for more research and information on the subject. It also raises several further issues including the need for an assessment of the health care requirements of the population, the allocation of resources and the setting of priorities, the importance of the evidence base of clinical practice, the need for clinical audit, and the problems surrounding the health care professional whose performance is poor.

The issue which affects the public most is that of variations in outcome from one hospital or one clinician to another. From the previous discussion it can be seen that there are many reasons for this disparity including the complexity of the cases (case mix) and the skills of the clinician. For example, many major hospitals are referred patients in a more advanced condition, and with unusual complicating factors in their diagnosis. It might thus be expected that such units might have poorer results, but for appropriate reasons. On the other hand there are variations which cannot be explained in this way and are identified as a result of clinical audit. It is for this reason that the setting of standards and monitoring of the outcome is so important and will be discussed later in other sections.

5. Evidence-based medicine

'Facts are Chiels that winna ding and downa be disputed'
Robert Burns

One of the important features of clinical practice is its grounding in science and evidence. Throughout medical school and postgraduate training the need to base decisions about patient care on scientific principles is emphasized. It is fitting therefore that the cause for 'evidence-based' or 'knowledge-based' medicine has been taken up by others and is seen to be a central part of the delivery of patient care. There are several different levels on which to assess the evidence. The first is through the randomized clinical trial in which a standard treatment is compared to a new or modified one and, by this method, over a period of years, the outcome is gradually improved. A good example of this would be the treatment of acute leukaemia in childhood, where, starting from a very low success rate in the early 1970s the use of clinical trials has improved the outcome enormously. While a very powerful method, especially if several trials can be combined in a meta analysis, they do have their drawbacks, and are not applicable in all conditions.

The second method is to use the evidence from studies carried out in carefully described groups of patients which, without a formal clinical trial being carried out, identifies improved treatment or diagnosis. This may be the starting point for larger trials of the procedure. The third method is to use a consensus of the 'great and the good' to determine, at a particular moment, what the best treatment might be. This is a very useful method when the illness may be treated in a variety of ways or in which the standard treatment has been in place for many years. Current textbooks of medicine and surgery represent much of this work, collected together. Indeed, the use of such resources as textbooks and audio visual material is an underrated method of setting out current practice. In a rapidly developing field, however, such methods may be too slow and rapidly outdated, although they remain a source of information and advice.

These three methods, alone or together, set the evidence base and the groundwork for the development of guidelines for good clinical practice. Such guidelines do no more than formalize clinical practice and set down in written form what would be the best course of action in particular illnesses. They should not be too tightly written so as to leave no room for individual clinical decision making and, more importantly, allowing the patient to make choices and be involved in the process. If guidelines become 'cook book' medicine they will have missed the point. They do however set standards against which practice can be assessed by the process of clinical audit. In all cases the guidelines will have a shelf life which will depend on the treatment and the disease. It is essential that they are updated regularly. They should not be seen as legally binding documents, but as *aides-mémoire* to good practice. The process of writing them and agreeing them within the team is in itself an educational experience.

As new treatments and diagnostic procedures become available they need to be assessed before they are introduced into clinical practice. The evidence for effectiveness should be set out before the development phase and introduction into routine use. This period, often described as health technology assessment, is an important part of the delivery of health care and links research, development, and clinical practice.

As an example of this process, the introduction of a new screening test for a common disease can illustrate the issues involved. Suppose a new test is suggested for a particular disease, and is subject to some pilot studies which indicate that it might detect the disease at an asymptomatic stage at which an intervention would eliminate the disease or change its natural history. The purpose of health technology assessment is to look carefully at the evidence, to seek expert views, and to come to a conclusion about the value of the test. Several options are possible, based on the evidence. First, that there is insufficient evidence, and that no further work need be done. Second, that the test might be useful but more evidence is required, or that targeting to a particular group may be necessary. Finally, the test may be assessed as so useful that it is recommended for introduction into clinical practice. Without such a process, ineffective treatments and procedures would be introduced leading to additional needless concern to patients and inefficient use of resources.

The evidence base therefore, together with the outcomes observed, should be part of the foundations of resource allocation in the health service—a subject which will be discussed later in this chapter.

6. Clinical audit

'Oh wad some power the giftie give us, to see ourselves as others see us.' **Robert Burns**

The need to review professional performance and to learn from the outcome is not a new issue in clinical practice. The 'audit' of the work carried out has always been part of good clinical practice. What is new is the recognition that clinical audit is an important tool for improving quality of care and, in addition, for fulfilling the understandable wishes of patients and managers to know that the quality of care is being regularly reviewed. The process of audit, the audit cycle, allows the objectives of care to be outlined, the action plan defined, the procedures implemented, and the results assessed. This last component, 'closing the audit loop', is critical as the outcome of audit should result in a confirmation that all is well, or more likely that things could continue to improve. Clinical audit therefore, defined as 'a systematic critical appraisal of the quality of clinical care, including procedures for diagnosis and treatment, the use of resources, and the resulting outcome and quality of life for the patient', brings together many of the components already discussed in relation to quality, clinical standards, and outcomes. This definition, emphasizing the clinical nature of the process, encourages teamworking and the sharing of the audit process.

Thus, clinical audit begins with a definition of the issue and the setting of standards. These standards can be national or local and should be based on the evidence of the effectiveness of the treatment, procedure, or diagnostic test. The implementation is planned and undertaken, and the results evaluated. It is the final part (closing the loop) which is of most significance, and the subject of most discussion. Once the results of the audit are available, what is to be done with them?

First, it should be noted that audit is about improving the quality of clinical care, and for that reason it would be expected that the results of audit will identify areas of clinical work which might need to change. That is the purpose of the process, there should be no concern about this. It is also why the process needs to be professionally led—to ensure that the results are credible and that action can then take place. If the process is seen as punitive (bad doctors doing poor work) then co-operation is likely to be less than it should. On the other hand, if it is seen in a positive way, as continually improving the quality of care, then it will be accepted and welcomed. Clinical audit is thus firmly associated with the process of education by which any deficiencies are remedied, and quality improved. It is crucial however that all practising clinical staff—doctors, nurses, dieticians, physiotherapists, and so on—take part. This is not a process for a few select people; it is for all staff.

The basis of the audit process is the setting of standards, generally agreed after discussions with the national professional bodies. For the process to be effective there is a need for supporting information systems to be available. One of the concerns is that the process, as just described, might stifle local initiatives or impede research. This must not be the case. Clinical audit is about the assessment of existing standards; research is about setting new ones which can then, if effective, be placed into the audit process. Local initiatives are in the same category. Such guidelines, subsequently audited, set a framework for good clinical practice. Local initiatives, if based on sound work, need not interfere with this process, and indeed should support it.

A further issue which is regularly raised is the question of the confidentiality of the results of audit. If the spirit of the process is agreed—that it is a way in which care can be continually improved—then the results of the process will be of particular relevance to the clinicians involved. Over the last 30 years, the Confidential Enquiries into Maternal Deaths (the first of its kind in the world), and the subsequent Enquiries into Postoperative Deaths and Deaths in Infancy, have shown how powerful the process can be. In general, the publication of such information to the wider world should go a long way towards increasing public confidence in the system, and assure the public and managers that the process is embedded in clinical practice. However, some issues arise with this approach which need further discussion. The first is that the results might show that an individual clinician, doctor, or nurse, is performing less well than would be expected. If this fact is then published, that individual has no opportunity to show improved performance by educational processes. If audit is about continual improvement, then it will be obvious that the baseline may vary. The second issue is the involvement of the public in the process. In England, the Clinical Outcomes Group (COG)—chaired jointly by the Chief Medical Officer and the Chief Nursing Officer—includes members of the public, specifically to assist in the audit process. It sends an important signal to audit groups around the country that such involvement is important. However it is not easy, and as is described in Chapter 4, there are few good models with which to work, and more innovative suggestions are required.

In most instances the process of audit will show how things can be improved, and the concerns just outlined, if handled sensitively, will result in more public confidence rather than less. It is in the few instances in which significant variations in outcomes are demonstrated that the real issues appear. If it is found that a nurse or a doctor fall far short of good practice, what should be done? This is a difficult subject which is discussed more fully in a later section of this chapter. Suffice it to say that the twin approach of prevention and regular feedback on performance, by for example mentoring, may assist with this. Local clinical governance is part of this process. The public do have a right to be sure about the quality of care, and it is the responsibility of all the professions to act rapidly on any issue which affects this confidence. Managers and the public have a right to be protected, and this will happen if the professions keep their own houses in order. Shakespeare had thoughts on this: 'How his audit stands who knows save heaven? But in our circumstance and course of thought, 'tis heavy with him.' *Hamlet*.

Clinical audit is thus a most useful tool to be used in improving the quality of care. It is not the only tool, but the professions must take it seriously if public confidence is to be maintained. The quality of care is excellent in this country, and the professions have little to fear and all to gain by supporting and ensuring that clinical audit is part of every professional's activity. In summary, the process should be:

- clinically led, recognizing the responsibilities involved
- seen as part of the educational process and part of routine clinical practice

- based on the setting of standards which are then followed through culminating in an assessment of the outcomes of care
- associated with the continual improvement in quality of care.

7. Maintaining professional standards: the role of mentoring

In all professions there are a few individuals whose performance and conduct is below that required by their profession. Estimating the total number is difficult but is likely to be between 2 and 5 per cent of the medical profession as a whole. The identification of such individuals is important not only from the point of view of public confidence, but also from the profession's interests. The medical profession, for example, is proud of its self-regulating status, and its ability to deal with problem doctors and to assure the public. Other professional groups also jealously guard their own standards. It is clear that each doctor or nurse has two professional responsibilities. The first is to ensure that their own professional practice is kept up to date, and that they regularly review the way in which it reflects standards. The second responsibility is to ensure that colleagues with whom they work are also maintaining such standards. If the figures given earlier are correct, then 95–98 per cent of staff are performing to a reasonable standard, but a small number are not. The mechanisms for ensuring standards have been covered elsewhere in this book and include clinical audit, regular programmes of continuing education, peer review, local clinical governance and exposure to wider professional views. In general this works well.

At the early stages of education at medical school there is a regular process of review and supervision. Defects in knowledge, skills, and attitudes can be identified and corrected. Similarly, during postbasic or postgraduate education, there are regular opportunities to review performance and to institute corrective measures. The problem lies at the career grade component of continuing education, where formal review occurs far less frequently. In general, the informal mechanisms already mentioned are sufficient—but clearly not in all cases. In addition, if a colleague is suspected of poor performance it may not be easy to discuss this. To assist with this, it is suggested that appraisal, peer review, or mentoring procedures are introduced. These allow for easier identification of problems and subsequent action. Where this has occurred, and is under way, it is seen as a very supportive programme in which learning is encouraged, good practice shared, and standards upheld and improved. Whether this needs to be followed up by some more formal processes is for discussion, but the public have a proper interest in the process. If the professions are to remain self regulating they will need to ensure that all steps are taken to assure the public.

8. Management and health services

There is a clear need to be able to manage health care and the resources which are provided for it. Management is important, and for many years it has not been given sufficient priority in the health service which has been undermanaged. But what is meant by management? First, it can be seen as a class of people, 'the bosses', who are in particular positions in an organization. Second, it may be regarded as a series of skills—strategic, personnel, finance, and so on. Or thirdly, management can be viewed as a series of values, held by senior members of the organization, and which set the tone and direction for the service. It is this latter definition which is considered most important, and the skills required follow from it. It links the management of the organization with the leadership required—a subject which is discussed elsewhere in more detail. Using this concept therefore, a manager is someone with a special set of values, who has the necessary skills to establish these values within the organization. Management style, as will be discussed later, may be less important. A key skill required is that of the handling of people—the heart of any organization. Without attention to staff and their welfare, the organization will not be as effective as it should be. All organizations are undergoing rapid change at the present. Without adequate input from staff at all levels, this process of change, instead of presenting opportunities, will be made more difficult than it need be.

Models of management

It is possible to construct several different models of management, each of which fit a particular organization or service. The first is what might be called the 'supermarket model', in which the head office sets the standards, does much of the purchasing, and defines the overall pattern of business. There are those in each of the stores who have some responsibilities for management, but this is within a framework set by the top. Those who are not managers of the store, but who have direct contact with the customer, have little freedom in the way they stack the shelves, serve the customers, and price the goods. In general, the skills at this end of the organization are limited, but are of great importance to each customer.

The second model is the 'operatic' one. In this model, the manager ensures that the production goes ahead and is of a high quality, facilitates the work of the conductor and the players, and makes sure that there is a programme which is responsive to the needs of the population. This model assumes that the public come to see the players, some of whom may be prima donnas and difficult to work with but have outstanding skills and talent. The conductor ensures that the performance is co-ordinated, and that the company work as a team, producing music of the highest quality. Everyone has a place, and the whole company works towards the same goal.

The third model can be described as the 'biological' model of management. It takes as its analogy the fact that humans and animals are able to manage themselves, to live, and to work in a most sophisticated way. Humans are remarkably responsive creatures, able to learn and adapt, to cope with enormous physical and mental demands, and yet, to continue to function. They have a huge capacity to store information, process it, and act accordingly. They are social animals, who need to take account of the environment in which they work. The model is a physiological one which draws on well-known principles of sensory perception, feedback loops, and action. It begins with the concept of intelligence and input from the senses, which keeps the organism in touch with the outside world. This is then synthesized and analysed by the brain, using the process of common sense. The body is composed of a series of organs, some capable of working and regulating themselves almost automatically, yet part of the whole. They have considerable autonomy. Feedback systems—neurological and endocrine—continually keep the head office (the brain) aware of what is going on so that central mechanisms can come into play as required. When internal action is needed, then there are several ways in which this can occur. External action, using the limbs or speech, allows communication and physical work to be done. It is a remarkable model, as the key feature is the brain, which allows thinking and creativity to be a central part of the organism. Without this, the organism would not be able to control part of its future. The brain plays the leadership role.

These three models are caricatures of what happens in real life, and within the health services. They do no more than stimulate discussion on what management is for, and how best it can be developed. What is not in doubt is the need to manage the skills and resources of the organization to achieve the best for the health of the population—the objective of the whole process.

The professions in management

Doctors, nurses, and other health professionals have an important role in management. First, they all have a responsibility for the way that they manage themselves, in terms of time and the use of their skills. Second, as part or leader of a clinical team, there is a responsibility to ensure that the resources are wisely used, and that the team works well and efficiently. As most health professionals will be in this category, they have a management role at this level in the organization. Some doctors and nurses have assumed a greater role in the management of the service—as a clinical director, medical director or chief executive. Generally, doctors make good managers. They are intelligent, clear thinking, with good diagnostic skills. They are accustomed to dealing with uncertainty, good with people, good communicators, and used to leading. The clinical skills of assessing a problem, identifying solutions, taking action, and reviewing the outcome, is simply the audit cycle, and part of clinical practice. They are used to using large databases, knowledge-based systems and networks, and in searching for solutions. Where they may need to enhance their skills often relates to their ability to think strategically, to look beyond their own specialty, and to develop financial expertise. Skills of selection and recruitment of staff are vital and at the heart of what managers do. They may also need to enhance their 'political' skills, though as Virchow said, 'Politics is just medicine writ large'. To do all this properly requires additional experience and training, and it is hoped that in the future management skills will become part of the medical curriculum at undergraduate and postgraduate levels.

Management style is perhaps less important than the ability to lead people in the right direction, and to transform them and the organization. It is about giving power to the staff and using their skills and resources. How this is done can therefore vary and depends on the issue. The 'contingency' theory of leadership (the ability to change style depending on the issue) may be the most flexible approach. Shakespeare contrasts two styles. The first—soft, encouraging, and supportive: 'Welcome hither; I have begun to plant thee and will labour to make thee full of growing.' *Macbeth* The second—harder and more decisive: 'If 'twere done then 'twere well it were done quickly.' *Macbeth*

Management and leadership are exciting tasks. Sir Roy Griffiths, who was instrumental in the UK in strengthening the management structure of the health service, used to say that the management of an organization required three things:

- quality assurance
- efficiency and the effective use of resources
- the motivation of staff.

If this is coupled with the view of John Kotter, in his book *The general manager*—'Great vision emerges when a powerful mind, working long and hard on massive amounts of information is able to see . . . interesting patterns and new possibilities' then the real excitement of the manager in improving the health of the population, and the health care provided, becomes evident.

9. Making choices: issues of resource allocation

It has always been necessary to make decisions about the use of resources for health and health services. Making choices is not a new concept, and neither are the issues which lie behind the difficulty in making them. The issues are essentially ethical and reflect the fact that resources are, and always will be, finite. Demand generally exceeds what is available, and the decisions made will allow some things to happen and others not. Until recently most of the decisions about resource allocation were made by the doctor, in relation to individual patients. As is discussed elsewhere, the consultation remains the basic building block of health care. However, this did result in some anomalies because some doctors were more successful (or their specialties more exciting to the public) than others in generating resources. The ethical issues involved have been discussed in Chapter 5, but boil down to the potential conflict between the individual rights of the patient (autonomy) and the needs of the population as a whole (utility). In making such decisions then, it is the value base of the organization which is the key factor. It is for this reason that public involvement in the debate is so important.

First, consider the use of the word 'resource'. This may be narrowly interpreted in terms of the funding available, or more broadly in terms of skills, facilities, and professional time. The second issue is how such decisions are made, particularly those which are concerned with slicing the whole cake of public expenditure, since it is not only the amount of money which goes to the 'health service' which is important, but also the funding and policies of the environment, education, transport, agriculture, and other government departments which will have an influence on health. Thus policy makers, with an interest in the 'health' of the population, need to think beyond the resources for 'health services'. That is the first, and perhaps most important level of decision making. The second level relates to the amount of resources for the 'health services' which are available, and the third is how these are then used effectively at the clinic or in the community. As resources are limited (in all countries) it is necessary to repeat again the fact that decisions need to be made about allocation, and that what is required is some basis for making the choices. In most circumstances the evidence required to make these decisions may not be adequate, and uncertainty about the outcome will remain. For this reason judgement is required, and this can be very difficult. What then might be the basic principles involved in recognizing this uncertainty, and the fact that at some point judgements have to be made?

The first principle is a consideration of the health and health service needs of the population. This establishes the baseline and should identify areas where investment in health care would have the maximum benefit. The techniques for doing this (assessing health gain) are available but need more work and refinement. The assessment of health need is a key public health function and should be able to delineate sections of the population, geographical areas, or particular diseases which require special attention.

The second principle is the ethical basis of decision making, taking into account issues such as justice, the rights and wishes of individuals, and the needs of the population as a whole. This can easily be illustrated by many recently publicized cases in which an individual or family wish treatment which is not only expensive but unproven, thus diverting resources from other areas. There is little point in arguing that 'more resources should be made available', because they have to come from somewhere. It is for this reason that there is a need to involve the public in these debates and to ensure that there is sufficient understanding of the problem and the process.

The third principle is to base the case for resource allocation decisions on the evidence available and only to fund those procedures which are effective. There is some evidence that a small amount of what doctors and other health care workers do results in little benefit. The amount of this is difficult to estimate, but identifying such ineffective clinical practice is one of the great professional challenges for the future. Because of the uncertainty about effectiveness, caution should be taken to avoid sweeping away much that is good. We are still at an early stage in the process of using evidenced-based medicine (in the way that it is now defined) as a basis for resource allocation.

If these three principles are followed (and there may be others), then there is the beginnings of a mechanism for decision making based on ethical principles and values, assessment of need, and evidence of quality of care and outcomes. This can be developed further to provide a framework for a comprehensive health service. At the end of the day however judgement will still be required to make resource allocation decisions. This topic is discussed further in Chapters 4 and 5, and issues of equity in Chapter 2.

A comprehensive health service

A framework can be developed which brings together much of the previous discussion. It is essentially a hierarchy of needs which become more and more sophisticated and more medically based. It extends from the responsibility of society to care for the population through to the need to evaluate new research-based interventions:

1. A caring society

It could be considered that all individuals in society have a right to be cared for. This does not imply that individuals have a right to treatment or to institutional care, but that in caring societies arrangements are made to ensure that those in need are provided with comfort and support. It is the principle of beneficence which is important, and the public recognition that to be cared for when required should be a basic value of society. Traditionally, this has been done within the family, with one or more members able to look after children, the disabled, the elderly, and the sick. As the structure of society changes this premise may need to be rethought.

2. Public health matters

All individuals should have access to a home; clean and safe water, air, and food; and access to evaluated and effective screening procedures. Immunization is the clearest example of this. As ill health can be related to the environment in the broadest sense, including communicable disease, this would be an important component.

3. Public education on health and health care

Many of the issues related to the provision of health services require public knowledge and understanding of health and skills in caring for the individual. As most of the care is delivered by individuals (more usually women, whose special role is discussed in Chaper 11), educational programmes need to be developed.

4. A primary care service

This is a fundamental part of a comprehensive service. It would include child health and maternity services, and provide individuals and their families with a front-line service to deal with the majority of illness and to ensure that health promotion is delivered. The UK is fortunate in having perhaps the best developed primary care service in the world.

5. Accident and emergency services
These provide for acute problems, including trauma. Life-saving measures are required to deal with such events and are a basic part of a comprehensive service.

6. Hospital-based services
These should deliver services whose value has been proven and based on sound evidence. Most can be gained from the use of procedures of known value, and the elimination of those whose outcome is poor. This must allow for the current state of knowledge, and not hinder research and development.

7. Expensive or special services
Such services or procedures (for example, heart transplantation, expensive diagnostic equipment) require to be planned on a population basis, at regional or national level.

8. New procedures to be evaluated on a research basis
In any comprehensive health service, research and development are essential and require careful planning, set within a framework of priorities for health care.

These eight points provide a general structure for health care. There may be many other ways of doing this, but it is hoped that this will once again stimulate discussion. Daniel Callaghan's book, *What kind of life*, sets out the issues in a similar way, developing them in a much more detailed way.

10. Information technology

Much of clinical practice is being transformed and improved by better and more effective means of information transfer. The use of computers is routine in many clinical areas, and it is not difficult to identify the ways in which this will continue—interactive technology, telemedicine, 'diagnosis at a distance', decision support systems, databases of ever increasing size and sophistication, and refinements to diagnosis and treatment. The use of IT networks can ensure that information and advice can be transmitted rapidly to anywhere in the world. Multimedia technology allows the use of film, graphics, and text to be available for improved clinical care. Record keeping and retrieval, ambulatory monitoring 'near-patient' testing, and many other uses all add to the vision of the revolution that IT can bring to clinical practice. But computers are only as good as those who develop them. In the words of T. S. Eliot:

> Where is the life we have lost in living
> Where is the wisdom we have lost in knowledge
> Where is the knowledge we have lost in information.

Thus there has to be a cautionary note sounded amongst the hype.

That said, the use of IT can genuinely help patient care. The portability of computers means that large databases can be available on the ward round or at the clinic. The facilities to check drug interactions, give information to patients, confirm the most up-to-date treatment available, and find the address of the local self-help group will all be possible. Evidenced-based medicine will become a reality as doctors and other health care workers review information and the reliability of the data. This will increase the role of the professional as it will allow greater interaction with the patient about the choices available, but will release him, or her, to spend more time with the patient dealing with questions and concerns and the difficult part of clinical work—communicating with the patient.

11. Communication

Throughout this book, the necessity for communication has been emphasized. Whether this is between patient and doctor, nurse and doctor, or doctor and the public, the theme remains important. Communication is a two-way process with sharing of information and ideas. It provides a channel through which one person's views and feelings can be described to another, with then an opportunity for response. Listening is a key element in good communication—active listening, creative listening, and other phrases have been used to describe the process. Generally, patients and the public tell us very clearly what they want to say. It is the professional's responsibility to listen and respond.

Being a two-way process, however, patients and the public also need to listen to the concerns and uncertainties of the doctor or the nurse. Denial is a very powerful coping mechanism, and several studies have shown that discussion of, for example, the diagnosis of an illness at certain stages, may not be fully understood by the patient; they miss key words and phrases. This problem needs to be recognized or even greater confusion can result.

Methods of communication

Communication between patient and doctor can take several forms. The simplest, but by no means the easiest, is verbal. This can be very difficult if the news is bad. The skills required are very special and take time, experience, and constant learning to acquire. No two problems are the same—each has to be discussed at the right pace, in the right environment, and at the right time. Sensitivity to the individual's views and feelings are paramount. The debate about telling the truth, and the need for individuals to know all of the facts, is a long one. There are no simple answers to these issues, other than the general principle that everyone has a right to know about their illness, its possible consequences, and treatment available. Only in this way can choices be made. But the process should proceed in a manner, and at a speed, which is comfortable for the individual. It also requires compassion, and in the words of St Bernard: 'Bitter is truth unseasoned by grace.'

A second method of communication is non-verbal, employing the use of body language. This can be remarkably powerful, as we show our feelings by our attitudes and demeanour. We may not need to say that all is not well to a patient, we can show it. A simple lack of courtesy, to failure to listen, or downright rudeness, all send messages to patients. On the other hand, warmth, friendliness, and treating people as people can be a very powerful way of cementing relationships.

Patients and families are the same. For both, body language, as well as what is said, can mean a lot. Dealing with a very ill relative can be difficult. Those who do this often say that they should be awarded an oscar for their acting ability—they appear bright, in control, say all the right things, and seem to be coping in front of their loved one; when alone however the fears and concerns surface.

The need to touch, and be touched, is a very powerful human need and essential part of body language. From the health professional's point of view, this closeness to the very ill patient is part of compassion. It is well described by Martin Buber in his book, *I and thou*, in which he relates two kinds of relationship. The first is the 'ordinary' type as between two strangers, where there is courtesy, respect, and a desire to help. This is the 'I and You' relationship. The second type, 'I and thou', is deeper. There is a 'sharing of hearts', which once established need not be mentioned, and indeed feelings and cares can remain unspoken as they are implicit in the relationship. Those who have experience of caring for seriously ill people will readily recognize this. It is one of the most fulfilling parts of a professional relationship and links to compassion and commitment to professional standards.

A third method of communication is to use the written or spoken word. This can be done in many ways—books to leaflets, audio tapes, videos, and electronically. On subjects which are of interest to specific groups, such as diabetes or osteoporosis, there can be enormously valuable input from those who have experience of and expertise in the problem, if we would only tap into it. Explanations of procedures, treatments, who the patient will see, follow-up, what to do and what not to do, and many other issues would all benefit by print or audio-visual presentations. These allow patients and their families to take time to reflect and to consider the kinds of questions which they want answered. If such information is given while the body language and words used by the professional indicate a willingness to listen and respond, then the conditions are right for effective communication.

One of the most beautiful stories about doctors, in the English language, is 'Rab and his friends' by Dr John Brown. It was written in the mid-nineteenth century, before the introduction of anaesthetics. The story is set in Edinburgh, and the hero is a young medical student, and Rab is a dog. The patient, Ailie, has breast cancer, and is due for an operation, which she subsequently undergoes, without anaesthetic, in front of the students—curtsying first to them. She subsequently develops an infection and dies. Before the operation she is seen by the 'great man', the surgeon. She asks 'when?' and he replies 'tomorrow'. As the medical student says, 'My master was a man of few words'. This small piece of communication can be interpreted in a number of ways, including as a clearly inadequate interaction, in which little information was given, no questions really answered, and certainly no choice provided for the patient. On the other hand, it could be that there was great trust in the relationship ('a sharing of hearts') and that little else was required. The story illustrates simply the complexity of the issues involved, and underlines the need not to assume that only one method of communication is correct.

The skill of communication

This leads to a brief discussion of the consequences of communicating the results of tests or treatments. If all is well then the process is relatively straightforward. It is when bad news has to be conveyed that the difficulties arise. As was said earlier, this is not easy and the effect of the bad news spreads outwards, like ripples, to the family and friends. The spreading ripples may also be reflected back to the patient, adding to the problem. To illustrate the point, a relative was once overheard to say 'It's alright for you, you've got cancer, I've got all the worries'. The therapeutic community—where the patient is being treated as part of the team—is a dynamic and powerful force for spreading the care, and ensuring that all concerned, including staff and patient, are looked after. We must not forget that staff are our most precious resource in health care and they need looking after too.

In his book, *Creative suffering*, Paul Tournier says that doctors (and by implication other members of the team) have two roles. The first is to do the best for the patient in treating and relieving symptoms. This is the traditional role of the doctor. The second is that the patient should be helped to benefit from his or her illness. This may seem a strange thing to say, but many will recognize the strength which can be found to cope with a difficult problem, enabling them to rise above the illness and indeed add new meaning to their life. This second role needs to be developed further.

Communication skills, however, are more than learning about the patient-professional relationship. To communicate well requires skills in advocacy for patients and the public; it is associated with presentational skills, in scientific meetings, and ward rounds; it needs the ability to chair meetings and deal with the media; it is a fundamental part of leadership. All of these must be considered and seen to be part of the process of becoming a professional.

12. Tales and legends in clinical practice

As one of the ways of linking education, research, and values within health care it is perhaps worth thinking about the role of tales and legends in clinical practice. Doctors, and other health professionals, learn in many ways, one of which is by listening to tales (case histories) about patients, diseases, and procedures. They tend to remember better the patient they have seen with a particular problem, than the page of a book they have read on the subject. Doctors are also very interested in medical legends—giants of the past or present who are admired and emulated. Tales are told about such legends, and the legends themselves usually excel in telling stories. Put a few doctors together and within a short space of time they reminisce about people and places, and there is enormous goodwill and fellowship in this process.

Joseph Campbell in his book, *A hero with a thousand faces*, makes the point that every culture in every time period requires heroes and legends—tales and stories of people and events which have taken the tribe (the medical staff) to greater and higher levels of skill and expertise. Often the hero has to face great difficulties, and goes through pain and suffering in the process, but at the end of the day the problem is solved, the dragon slain. The sagas fill in the long winter evenings (continuing medical education) and inspire young men and women to try even harder. They boost morale, and are part of the leadership process. Howard Gardner in his book, *Leading minds*, emphasizes the importance to leaders of being able to tell convincing stories which will encourage others to follow. The most difficult task however, is to tie these tales and legends to the mainstream of clinical practice. Tales can be misleading, legends less than perfect, and there needs to be standards and reference points which give credibility to the individual case history or the attitudes and skills of a particular doctor. In other words, how far are these individual tales and legends representative of clinical practice as a whole?

Some personal examples might help to illustrate this further. I can vividly remember individual patients, clinical signs, and even the bed or room the person was in. This is not unusual. I can clearly recall being taught a particular way to palpate the abdomen by a senior surgeon who had a lightness of touch and superb diagnostic skills. Patients with particular symptoms, pain for example, are easily recollected. Family issues, grief, loss, and recovery are vividly brought to mind. I have always been fortunate in the people I have worked with—men and women of real stature—and have no difficulties in recounting tales about their clinical and non-clinical skills. As a medical student I recall a senior professor who was able to take the pulse, blood pressure, and temperature with one hand in a few seconds. Not the only way to do it—but memorable. Colleagues who provide a painstaking clinical opinion in a difficult clinical area, and surgical skills of the highest quality are the bedrock of British medicine.

But, how does one know that the tale or the legend holds true? How does one connect personal experience with that in clinical practice as a whole? How does one know that one's special tale (case history) is representative of the generality of patient care? This is the key. Learning by personal experience is a very powerful way of gaining new knowledge and changing practice and behaviour, but it needs to be placed in context. Several methods have evolved over the years to help with this:

1. **Telling the story to someone else**
This is particularly helpful if it is a long and difficult saga, when a wise person with considerable experience can help to interpret the signs. This is known as a consultation. A great deal can be learned by this kind of problem-based interaction by an expert.

2. **Telling the tale to several others**
The use of seminar case presentations or 'grand rounds' provides an opportunity to set the individual problem in a broader context. This may be done by the doctor in a search of the research literature, or by having others at the scene of the storytelling who have a wider experience. This process is also valuable for allowing the perfection of the art of storytelling (case presentation).

3. **Moving between legends**
One of the strengths of British medical educational programmes, is the ability to move between clinical units and to be exposed to new thoughts and tales. This allows comparisons to be made and enables the true legend to be identified—a very important process.

4. **Linking with the literature**
The individual problem encountered in the clinic can be put into perspective by a review of the journals—printed or electronic. How often does that side-effect generally occur? Is this the usual age of presentation? How regularly is treatment effective? All can be answered by tales told many times before and collected together as a review of the literature.

5. **Creating a new tale**

Many of the clinical issues identified in the course of practice will not be new and will have been described before, perhaps with greater clarity and style. Really exciting is the telling of a completely new story, from an idea or an observation which is original and different. This puts one directly into the 'legendary' category, particularly if at the same time one can solve the problem. Curiosity and the need to see and do new things (research) is a fundamental part of being a doctor.

6. **Leadership and telling stories**

Leadership is one of the most important aspects of medicine, and other professional groups at the present time. Leaders tend to be those about whom stories are told, and who themselves lead by communicating their vision. They can simply, clarify, and tell the tale in a way which assures that others will follow. Other aspects of the subject of leadership will be discussed in a subsequent section.

13. Memories: a neglected concept in care

Some personal reflections

It is surprising sometimes how a series of chance events, comments, or ideas set off a train of thought that leads to a rethinking of patterns of care provided for patients, families, and staff. A few lines from a television programme and a comment from a relative and a patient, occurring within a few hours of each other, occasioned my review of the concept of memories. As usual, the concept is not new, but its importance in the provision of care is perhaps sufficiently neglected for us to remind ourselves of the implication of memory. Nor is the recognition of the importance of memories a new one. Their psychological significance is well recognized, and for professionals our experience and recollection of events, people, or incidents affect our clinical practice and are an important stimulus to learning. Neither is it a surprising concept. Talk to any group of patients, relatives or friends, or colleagues about an event involving medical care and the phrase, 'I remember . . .', occurs frequently. What was new for me was the implication behind the statement, for the quality of care delivered. These random thoughts, therefore, led me to take a closer look at 'memories' in clinical care.

The first thought that struck me was that memories are uniquely related to the individual and sometimes bear little relation to what actually happened. They are often intensely personal and tiny details of what happened, of which others may have taken little or no notice, may stand out. It is not possible to predict what will be remembered by any individual, and this idiosyncrasy is crucial to the concept of memory and its place in the provision of care. The link with learning is relevant here too. Faced with almost any critical situation (a sick child, a patient in coronary care, a postoperative problem), a group of medical students will, individually, recollect and learn different aspects from these cases. So it is with patients and relatives. The personal, individual view predominates. Inevitably, if one sees patients who are ill or dying many of the events remembered relate to the period of the last illness. The lessons learned, however, are applicable to all aspects of medicine and all episodes of care.

The second thought was that memory covered several different, though related, activities. There is the memory of the doctor and what he or she said or did; of the place of care—ward, room, house; and of the patient and the family, and their response to the illness. It is not uncommon for the doctor or nurse to remember particular places, rooms, or their furnishings associated with an individual patient, long after the patient has gone. It is not difficult to recollect how a doctor dealt with a member of the family. Specific memories are important, as is their impact. For example, one nurse recalled the arrangement of flowers outside a particular ward which reminded her of a funeral parlour. She could not enter the ward without thinking about this. In contrast, other nurses felt that the area was welcoming and friendly. The memory of the kindness of the nurse, a smile, a handshake, a word of thanks a telephone call can often be instantly brought to mind.

Then there is the memory of the illness itself and the specific effects of it on the patient and the family. The 'ripple' effect can be extensive and long lasting. How often have we heard the statement (or something similar) from a patient or relative currently under care, 'My father had cancer 20 years ago, and we had a terrible time looking after him'? These memories are retained and talked about. They become part of the folklore and culture, and condition families to expect a certain kind of care and outcome. If the care and outcome had been different, how would this have affected the memories? For a doctor or nurse, the memory of a death, especially if it occurred early in training, can have a major, long-term influence on the perception of the dying. This can be positive, encouraging a more active approach and a desire to do better. Or it can be negative, making the doctor or nurse avoid contact with such patients in the future. Another example might illustrate this more clearly: one poor response to chemotherapy, one toxic reaction, can have a profound effect on the caring team, never mind the relatives or patient. In discussion, several general practitioners have said how they remembered as house officers giving 'cytoxics' to patients who were dying. These memories left a lasting impression and clearly coloured their views on the treatment of cancer. For other illnesses and treatments, the analogies are pertinent. It emphasizes the need for careful explanation and support of staff when new or potentially hazardous treatment is to be given. Memories, rational or not, can be of good events or bad events. For the relatives, memories may be the thing that they hold on to once their loved one has gone—memories of things said or done together, or with the professional team. Bitterness can remain for a very long time and can override the pleasant memories of years of happiness. Alternatively, if the last memories are good, they can wipe out previous problems.

In practical terms, therefore, we can be sure that memories are important. But what can be done to ensure that they carry with them positive, rather than negative reactions? It is necessary to recognize that memories are part of the system of patient care, whether we like it or not. Memories are about small things as well as big events, and for this reason attention to detail is important. Putting yourself in the place of the patient or relative and asking what kind of memory you would like to retain from the situation can be salutary.

When working with colleagues of whatever professional group, it is useful once again to ask the question, 'What will they remember about this patient, this illness, or the attitude of staff?' I can still remember the first very ill young patient I had to look after as a houseman, and the support I was offered by senior staff. Kindness of senior members to juniors is always remembered. For relatives, the last few days and weeks they live with their loved ones may be the time, out of decades of a relationship, they remember best. The good times are forgotten and overtaken by the events of the last few hours. As members of the caring team it is our responsibility to ensure that these memories are as positive as possible. To do this it is necessary to look and listen and be sensitive to the needs of others. Our own memories are also important—memories of colleagues, patients, friends, hospitals and homes, episodes of illness, and unusual responses. Memories are long lasting and require careful nurturing, and should be built with the care we give to patients, families, and colleagues.

If it is quality of care which we wish to deliver, then it is attention to detail which deserves special effort.

Further reading

Buber, M. (1958). *I and thou.* SCM Press, Edinburgh.

Callaghan, D. (1995). *What kind of life: Limits to medical progress.*

Campbell, J. (1949). *The hero with a thousand faces.* Princeton University Press.

Gardner, H. (1995). *Leading minds. An anatomy of leadership.* Basic Books, New York.

Tournier, P. *Creative Suffering.* SCM Press, Edinburgh.

11

Some special issues in health care

1. Introduction

Throughout this book some issues of particular concern to health care have been identified. They include the developments which will occur as we look ahead to the new millennium (Chapter 13), and some of the health care issues in developing countries (Chapter 9). This chapter brings together a few topics which, although already mentioned, deserve further emphasis.

2. Primary care

This is the heart of most health care systems. In the UK, the primary care led National Health Service is not just a slogan, but a clear statement of its importance. Primary care is in the front line of the health service. The general practitioner acts as the gatekeeper to secondary and tertiary care, providing a wide range of services including early diagnosis, preventative advice, treatment,and follow-up. The primary care team act as the advocate for the patient, co-ordinating the care provided and guiding him or her through the health care journey. This requires teamwork and a range of skills and expertise—medical, nursing (in all its diversity), pharmacy, and, increasingly, public health practice.

There is now greater emphasis on health as well as illness. The primary care team work, generally, with a defined population and are therefore able to assess the health needs (not just the medical needs) of patients and the population as a whole. Recent developments in information technology have allowed more effective methods of call and recall, and provided useful, confidential databases for the purpose of audit. Thus, individuals or groups with special needs can be more effectively identified and managed. Finally, the advent of telemedicine provides a link between the general practitioner, or one of the team, with the specialist services.

The primary care team offer long-term care for patients and, over a period of years, are able to care for indiviudals and families. The general practitioner is therefore seen as a personal doctor to the patient and not only to be available at times of crisis. This personal link is very important for the purposes of health promotion, protection (as in immunization), and prevention.The team also have an excellent opportunity to involve the patient and the public in decision making. As much health care is self-care, the situation is favourable for patient education, and in helping patients to understand symptoms and disease processes.

If we did not have primary care we would need to invent it.

3. Mental health

In all countries and all cultures mental health issues are of great concern, partly because of the numbers of people who may be affected, but also because of the stigma associated with mental illness. The range of illness varies from relatively minor problems of anxiety or depression to major problems of psychotic disease. Environmental influences such as violence, war, unemployment, the breakdown of a social network, and interpersonal problems can all affect the quality of life of individuals and families. There are important links to the criminal justice system, and to substance abuse with alcohol or drugs.

All age groups have mental health problems. In children they often relate to learning difficulties or behavioural problems. In adolescence, issues of personal identity and experimentation with different lifestyles and behaviours are relevant. In young men, in many parts of the world, there are problems of suicide and violence; and in the elderly, the difficulties of loneliness and dementia. Bereavement issues are often forgotten and, at a time of need, their special problems overlooked. The scale of the problem is substantial. In any one year, for example, there will be over 600 000 individuals with dementia in England.

Culturally, most people find it easier to deal with physical problems rather than mental ones. Perhaps this is not surprising as they are psychologically often too complex to explain on a rational basis. Yet the stigma surrounding mental illness makes it all the more difficult to talk about and hence to help those in need. In this regard, carers need special mention. They perform a remarkable job, sometimes without any acknowledgement, in caring for their loved ones. The setting of care has also changed significantly, moving from the large Victorian asylums to community or home-based care. Quality of life issues are paramount.

For the future it will be necessary to try to remove the stigma of mental illness, and to increase public understanding and involvement in the problems. There is also a need to recognize the important links between the environment and mental health.

4. The elderly

As health care improves and medical advances change the way disease can be managed, so the population lives longer. This phenomenon is occurring in all countries. As the numbers rise, the issues are compounded by changing family and social structures. The link to social care is obvious. As the numbers of older people in the population rise, so it is important to ensure that their quality of life is not diminished. Hence the equal importance of health promotion in this age group. For example, regular exercise and an adequate diet can modify the risk of developing a fracture from osteoporosis and, at the same time, promote well-being. As the illnesses are often of a degenerative nature, such as is the case with arthritis, maintaining mobility and self-care not only reduces symptoms but allows contact with others to be kept up, thus minimizing the threat of loneliness. Social isolation is a major problem. Older people have much to give and they need to be well enough to give it. A great deal can be done by appropriate assessment of need and the planning of care.

The long-term care of the elderly is receiving attention around the world. Many different models have been assessed and used. The Royal Commission recently set up in this country is an important step in analysing the issues which face us all.

5. Adolescence

This is a period of life in which there is rapid growth and change. It is characterized by experimentation and challenging authority. In the words of Shakespeare:

> I would there were no age between ten and three and twenty, or that youth would sleep out the rest; for there is nothing in the between but getting wenches with child, wronging the ancientry, stealing and fighting—Hark you now!

Little has changed over the years. Adolescence is a time when behavioural patterns are set and during which there are substantial bodily changes culminating in physical and sexual maturity. Passage through this leads to adulthood and responsibility. It is therefore an imoprtant time during which the combined influence of the environment and culture on the one hand and health messages on the other strive for ascendency. The outcome determines, at least for a period of some years, the lifestyle of the young person.

From the point of view of the health service it is a time when special provision may be required, particularly for those with chronic diseases such as cystic fibrosis, asthma, the cancers, and diabetes. They may be being cared for in a children's setting or an adult one, and neither may be appropriate. The sensitivity which is experienced about body image and feeling abnormal can be especially acute. For this reason the provision of dedicated facilities should at least be considered.

6. The health of men

Men's health is generally poorer than women of the same age. Women live longer, a fact which has been known for many years. Typically, men are not as concerned about their health and do not seek medical attention as readily as women; they present with illness later than they might, and they do not talk as openly about their problems as women (which might, in part, be associated with the higher incidence of suicide in younger men). While in most age groups the age specific mortality is falling, that of the 15–40 year-old male is rising. This is a tragic loss of young lives. The causes are mainly due to violence, injury, and self-harm—alcohol and drugs playing an important part in this. Coronary heart disease rates and lung cancer rates are particularly high, though falling. Of the specific problems of males, testicular cancer now has a very good prognosis if treated early, while prostatic disease, both benign and malignant, presents major health care problems.

Perhaps less attention than might have been was focused on men's health in the past. In recent years this has changed, and there are now more innovative programmes available to improve their health.

7. The health of women and the role of women in health

One of the themes of this book has been that women are central to improving health. Women are the principle carers and they have a particular concern for the health of children and families. They make choices about diet and have a substantial influence on lifestyle and behaviour. The level of educational attainment of women is also important—the higher the level, the better the health. It is women who generally make the diagnosis within the family and are likely to be the person who begins treatment or recommends that a health professional gives an opinion. The 'wise woman' has an important part in the health of the community, though 'old wives tales' may not always be the best way of dealing with illness.

The illnesses which are specific to women relate to various disorders of the female genital trace and the breast. Pregnancy and childbirth are normal events but in some parts of the world these remain hazardous. Under age pregnancy is a particular problem. Many of the health problems of women relate to culture and social issues including violence and any restrictions in human rights and liberty. Discrimination remains a major factor.

It has been suggested by some with whom this book has been discussed that too much prominence has been given to the role of women. It is true that family life is very much a partnership with the sharing of time and experience. That is correct, and where it exists then men, in relation to the health of the family, are equally important. Where it does not, then the argument still stands.

8. Disability

A very wide range of physical, sensory, and psychological disabilities occur in the population. These include hearing, sight, mobility, and neuromuscular disorders. The levels of seriousness of disability increase with age, and there are often multiple forms of disability in the one person. The numbers involved are large:

1. 18 per cent of males and females over 16 years have moderate or severe disability.
2. More than 60 per cent of over 60 years old and more than 70 of over 85 years old have disability.

3. 40 per cent of reported causes of disability in children are related to diseases of the ear and mastoid.
4. Accidents cause 7–27 per cent of all disabilities.
5. 7 per cent of men and 11 per cent of women have a bladder problem; 34 per cent of women over 75 years use an incontinence pad.

Each needs special care and attention, and the recognition that their needs will be met. Discrimination, in any form, has to be tackled positively. Access is a particular problem and limits activity and reduces quality of life. People with disability have much to offer society, and they can and should be able to enjoy life. A recent poster shows a physically disabled young man rock climbing in a wheelchair with the caption 'Can't is a four letter word'. Given the opportunity, the potential can be realized.

9. Rehabilitation

In the search for better and more effective treatment, perhaps even cures, the role of rehabilitation can easily be forgotten. It is strongly linked to issues of quality of life and well-being. The process begins, as always, with an assessment of need, and a definition of a plan, agreed with the patient, to restore physical and mental health. This requires the skills of many health professionals including physiotherapists, dieticians, occupational therapists, and speech therapists. The range of problems is enormous, from rehabilitation after a heart attack or stroke, to that required following major trauma. It includes both physical and psychological rehabilitation after breast cancer, or that following a mental illness. Teamwork is essential to make use of the full range of skills required. But rehabilitation is more than that. It is a philosophy, a concept, which should be integral to all clinical practice: it is about helping the patient to return to a full and active life, or if that is not possible, to help them to achieve all that they can.

10. Health in the workplace

Most of us spend a considerable amount of our lives at work. For those interested in health it is an appropriate setting within which to provide a healthy environment. Safety in the work environment is paramount and must be taken seriously. But, additionally, the workplace can provide healthy eating, facillities for exercise, social contact, and help and advice when required (the availability of counselling for alcohol and drug problems would be part of this). Stress is part of life, but excess psychological pressure can lead to serious consequences. A good employer will recognize the problem and set up mechanisms to deal with it proactively. A healthy workforce is a good workforce, and good health is good business.

Occupational health can sometimes be seen as being not as important as dealing with acute problems or carrying out research. Yet to neglect the health of the workforce is a short-sighted agenda. Human resources—the people who work with you—are the most valuable resources available. Their well-being is as important to the employer as it is to the employee.

Those who are not in work also have special problems. In most instances the mortality and morbidity in this group are higher than the population as a whole. There are many possible reasons for this, but what is clear is that those who are unemployed have particular health problems which require as much care and compassion as those in work.

11. Conclusions

The topics described in this chapter are only a few of those that might have been chosen, but they serve to illustrate the breadth of care and to emphasize the need to think widely and not to forget important groups, even though their voice might be weak. The overriding principle of equity should ensure that this does not occur.

12

Professional issues

'Knowledge must always precede reformation.' **Thomas Muir**

1. Introduction

This chapter brings together several interlocking themes, each of which emphasizes the role of the professions in improving the health of the population. The model chosen is the medical profession—its educational foundations, its values and ethical base. The issues for other professional groups are similar, and interrelated, and lessons can be learned from each other. To stress this point there is a section on teamwork and interprofessional education.

The first part of the chapter deals with the role of the profession of medicine. This is an area of considerable public interest. What are doctors for? How should they be regulated? What is their role in health as opposed to illness? This inevitably leads to a consideration of values and the ethical principles of a profession. This is done by looking critically at the Hippocratic Oath and its relevance to medicine as we approach the twenty-first century. The aim is to draw out some of the questions raised by such a consideration and open up the debate. Finally, the chapter discusses educational issues for doctors and other professional groups.

Perhaps at this stage there is a need to say more about the justification for a chapter with this title in a book about health. There are several reasons, which have already been raised in Chapter 1. First is the need to shift the thinking of professionals and the public from illness to health. That cannot be done without the commitment of doctors and other health professionals. The second is that professional leadership is an important component (others include political and public leadership) of improving health and achieving the potential. Thirdly, if we are to change the knowledge base, improve outcomes, maintain a critical and evaluative attitude in health professionals, then this needs to be built into the educational process. Education (as will be discussed later) is a lifelong process; professional education is an important key to changing and improving health.

2. The profession of medicine

There is increasing public and professional interest in medicine, with questioning of professional standards and the quality of care provided. Public expectations of the level of service to be delivered are rising. It is timely therefore to review the role and purpose of medicine, and the concept of a profession.

At the outset it should be clear that the medical profession in this country provides a service to individuals and the population which is the envy of the world, and the commitment within the National Health Service to maintain this is real and deeply held. Because of this the profession had nothing to fear by being open and encouraging debate on how services could be even better. And that is the thread which goes through this chapter. Doctors and other professionals provide one of the most valued public services in this country, and are held in high esteem. However, this will only continue to be the case if they take the lead in promoting change and improvement—in other words, to consider their role as a profession.[1,2,3]

What is the purpose of medicine?

The purpose of medicine is to serve the community by continually improving health, health care, and quality of life for the individual and the population, by health promotion, prevention of illness, treatment and care, and the effective use of resources—all within the context of a team approach. This emphasizes a series of key issues; a focus on patients, health and quality of life, the use of resources and the team approach; which will now be discussed in more detail.

What is a profession?

It is not easy to define a profession but it is likely to have some or all of the following characteristics:

(1) it is a vocation or calling and implies service to others
(2) it has a distinctive knowledge base which is kept up to date
(3) it determines its own standards and sets its own exams
(4) it has a special relationship with those that it serves—patients, clients
(5) it has particular ethical principles—the ethical base
(6) it is self-regulating and is accountable to patients or clients, and to the profession itself.

Each of these is essential for ensuring public confidence in medical practice, and in retaining credibility. From each can be derived further, or secondary principles and values in medicine, such as the importance of continuing education, quality, and the role of research and development. Changing the culture and ethos of the health service has sharpened the focus on the value base of medicine. These principles, or similar ones, are crucial, and are not dependent on the organization and structure of the health service. They require wide debate.

What do doctors do?

This question is broadly about the role of medicine, although it can also refer in a more restricted way to the particular contribution of clinical practice. In turn, it also tries to answer the question 'what do doctors do that others don't?' Clearly, doctors see patients, do investigations, prescribe or carry out treatment, do research, and teach.

They care for patients and this aspect, which includes commitment and compassion, is very important. This aspect, together with the skills required to do it well must not be undervalued. Some doctors care for whole families, or whole communities, and bring to them the same kinds of skills and expertise. But it could be said that other professional groups do many of the same things. Doctors have no monopoly of caring, investigations, research, or even treatment—though there remain many forms of treatment which are only carried out by doctors.

However, there is one profoundly important aspect of practice which is generally carried out by doctors, and that is in making a diagnosis and in assessing its consequences. The implications of this are crucial. The consultation, the accumulation of information, the making of a diagnosis, and the setting out of the prognosis and possible treatment, are the basic building blocks of health care and resource allocation. Further, a key part of this is the communication of the diagnosis, prognosis, and treatment to the patient or community. Making a diagnosis is not simple and straightforward, even when the name of the 'disease' is well recognized. Social and family implications are critical, emphasizing the holistic nature of the concept and of patient care. It is a person with an illness, not just a label, and the wider implications of the 'diagnosis' need stressing. The making of a diagnosis through history taking, physical examination, and investigation is also very important, and should not be fragmented into a series of unrelated processes. A systematic approach is necessary. Clinical skills are, after all, still fundamental to medical practice. At this stage others may take the lead role in following through with treatment, counselling, and so on, but the essential issue remains the diagnosis, its communication, and the setting out of a plan of action (agreed with the patient or the community) on the management of the problem.

This raises a further issue as to what is meant by a diagnosis, and what are its dimensions. This can clearly range from a provisional working hypothesis through to histopathological confirmation. In each instance there are likely to be uncertainties, and one of the skills of the craft of medicine is to be able to communicate these. Learning to live with uncertainty as a patient is not easy, and, as the disease process evolves, continuing support and explanation is required. However, this emphasizes again the central nature of the diagnosis, its consequences in health care, and the need for an holistic approach.

In most instances it is the diagnosis which will determine the resource required (in some instances the patient will, quite properly, not wish the treatment). It is the technology which will further define that resource. This may be surgical treatment, a medication, physiotherapy, a special diet, counselling and so on—the range is enormous. As the technology changes, so the resources will vary, and the rate of change in clinical practice is increasing every year. This means that doctors must keep up to date and be sure that new treatments are worthwhile before they are widely introduced, emphasizing the role of research and development, education, and of outcome assessment. These issues will be discussed further.

Doctors also have responsibilities for the use of resources. This should not be narrowly defined in terms of funding, though this is important, but should also include the appropriate use of time, skills, and available facilities. A doctor who spends two hours with one patient, cannot spend these hours with another. Similarly, if a sum of money is spent on one patient, it will not be available for another. Resources are, and always have been, finite. The classical dilemma of the doctor is how to do the best for one patient, without disadvantaging another. The fact that this is difficult must not mean that doctors abrogate their responsibilities. Central to this is an understanding of the outcome of care, and the ability to make such difficult judgements on the basis of knowledge and evidence. Trust is a key element in this process. It may be necessary to separate decision making at the bedside from resource allocation at a higher level.

Thus doctors could be seen to have three broad roles—firstly, to provide high-quality care, and in particular to be concerned with diagnosis, prognosis, treatment, and the planning of care and the communication of this to the patient; secondly, to be interested in the individual and the community; thirdly, to manage resources—including skills, time, facilities, and finance—effectively. Combined with a view from the perspective of the patient, these roles should give a complete picture. The purpose of the doctor can then be refined as answering the following series of questions:

1. What is wrong with me?—the diagnosis.
2. What does this mean for me?—the prognosis.
3. What can be done for me?—the caring and management component.
4. What can I learn from this patient?—the research dimension.
5. How can others benefit?—the public health dimension.
6. What can I teach others from this experience?—the educational opportunities both for patients and professionals.

What kind of doctor do we need?

If we agree as to the purpose of medicine, what a profession is, and what doctors do, it becomes possible to consider the kind of doctor we need. This is far from easy, as a consideration of the range of specialties identifies several characteristics. Is it possible therefore to describe a core of characteristics, for all doctors? The following section includes what can best be classified as key values expected of all doctors—independent of the specialty, and indeed independent of the structure and organization of the health service. But first an illustration.

Heberden–a case study All of us have our heroes. Mine include the Hunter Brothers (William and John), Thomas Sydenham, Sir William Tennent Gairdner, Sir William MacEwan, Sir William Osler, Sir George Newman, and a number of my contemporaries (who will not be identified for fear of embarrassing them). One of the most important figures is Dr Heberden. He lived between 1710 and 1801, at a fascinating time in the history of medicine, with the eighteenth century showing significant advances in the practice of medicine and in the understanding of disease. It is said that Dr Samuel Johnson in his last illness called for 'Dr Heberden, ultimus romanorum, the last of our learned physicians'. He exemplified three important attributes of the doctor: he was a clinician, a scientist, and a scholar. As a clinician he was highly respected, and much sought after. As a scientist he made important original observations, all clearly written up. As a scholar he had interests beyond medicine, and was noted for his wisdom and learning. These may not be on everyone's list of attributes, but they express some values to which to aspire.

Key 'values' expected of doctors

1. **High standard of ethics**

From the time of the Hippocratic Oath, medical practice has always had a very strong ethical foundation, and rightly so, as it is one of the key features of a profession. More than ever the ethical principles associated with clinical practice need to be debated and clarified. New procedures and ethical dilemmas arise constantly. Greater public awareness of the issues (and it is appropriate that the wider public are involved) means that the debates are no longer confined to professional audiences. There is greater scrutiny of professional practice, and standards are now openly discussed in the press and public forum. The profession has nothing to fear from such debates as long as it is not defensive or secretive.

2. **Continuing professional development**

This concept (which is broader than continuing education, which will be discussed later) is concerned with personal growth and satisfaction with professional work. It is an area which has been neglected in recent years but, with the changing role of the consultant, it is one which will need to be looked at afresh in the near future.

3. **The ability to work in a team**

As medicine and health care increase in complexity, so it becomes even more necessary to be sure that all the skills of professions other than medicine are utilized to the full. This means working and learning in teams, but it does not mean relinquishing the key patient-doctor relationship which is so central to the therapeutic process.

4. **Concern with health as well as illness**

Are doctors only to be concerned with those who are ill, or do they have a wider role in the community in preserving health?

5. **Patient and public focused**

The purpose of medicine, if you agree with the definition given earlier, is precisely to do with serving the patient and the public. Perhaps we should be more willing to say this explicitly, rather than implicitly. There is great energy and power in this process if it can be harnessed effectively.

6. **Concern with clinical standards, outcomes, effectiveness, and audit**

More and more of the care given to patients, and the treatment offered, will be based on proper outcome-based evidence. This is not to deny innovation, or to stifle research and development. Rather the opposite. Standards record where we are now; research and innovation should take us to new levels of quality and care. It is clear from many studies that there are variations in treatment and outcomes across the country. Some of these are understandable and explainable; others are not. It is this aspect, which from a public and professional point of view, requires resolution. Audit is a tool which has value in measuring the quality of care provided. It is only one tool, but an essential one to assure quality. As part of professional practice, all doctors should be involved in auditing clinical work.

7. **Ability to define outcomes**

Outcomes, in some instances, are not easy to define, though this is an important professional challenge. The use of guidelines—which can be seen as no more than the formalization and clarification of good clinical practice—is part of the process of care, and not an end in itself. The guidelines need to be feasible, to encourage local involvement, and not to inhibit new methods of management; rather to be a base on which to build. They should help us to understand and explain variations in care.

8. **Interest in change and improvement, research, and development**

Medicine cannot, and should not, stand still. It is continually evolving and improving. All doctors need to be involved in changing and improving clinical practice, indeed they have an obligation to do so, though this does not mean that all need to participate in 'research'. It emphasizes however the importance of academic input and of teaching.

9. **Ability to communicate**

Of all the complaints against doctors, failure of communication must be one of the most frequent. Yet it is perhaps a central role of the doctor if you accept that making a diagnosis, assessing prognosis, and defining treatment are key elements of his or her work. Arrogance and discourtesy reflect badly on a profession whose primary purpose is to care for patients. The importance of communication as a two-way process is being increasingly recognized in medical schools, and role models (consultants and GPs) must also acknowledge the effect of the 'hidden agenda' (their attitudes and behaviour) on medical students and postgraduates.

What are the implications of these questions?

Some of the implications have already been discussed, others will be picked up now:

1. **Medical education: the knowledge base and the curriculum**

This is a most important issue. We must see medical education as a continuum that includes continuing medical education (CME), and recognize that doctors have an ethical obligation to keep up to date. Understanding the knowledge base is part of being a professional, and needs to constantly be updated and replenished. There is much to be said about education and training, but here only one further point will be made, and that is to distinguish between the two concepts. To be trained is to have arrived; to be educated is to continue to travel. Doctors must have a broad vision of the world, and be able to change and adapt as the knowledge base changes. They need to have outside interests, and be rounded people, with breadth as well as depth.

2. **Public involvement**

This is easy to say but difficult to carry out. Who are the public, and how can we best obtain their input? Perhaps the best solution is to be much more specific, and to select the public or patient group to fit the issue. These issues are discussed further in Chapter 4.

3. **Quality**

Quality is difficult to define, both at an individual practitioner level and at the level of a clinical unit. A question which is commonly asked relates to how it might be possible to measure quality in a clinical unit. Some suggestions are given in Chapter 10.

4. **Theoretical base**

Models of health and disease are required to provide a foundation for progress. The development of general theories of health and illness would help to underpin the understanding of disease and the maintenance of health. (See Chapter 1.)

5. **Doctors in management**

This is a major issue at present, and one with which the profession must come to terms. Do doctors wish to be involved in management, and if so at what level? Clearly they should be involved in managing patients, their own time, and the resources at their disposal. But what of the tasks beyond that—as clinical directors, medical directors, chief executives, general managers? Not all doctors will wish to be involved at all levels, but the profession must consider carefully the opportunities, be able to take them, and support those who do.

6. **Leadership and vision**

These are certainly important attributes and more than ever we need them in the senior members of the profession. We must be able to look beyond the present and to identify where we would like to be, and the kind of values which are necessary. A recent book, *Learning to succeed*, says in one of its chapters, 'education is the process by which values are transmitted from one generation to another'.[2] We must be sure of what the values are and develop strategies to attain them. The role of the teacher in this is crucial.

7. **Professional organization and self-regulation**

One issue which surfaces increasingly is the organization of the profession, and its need to remain self-regulating. Under increasing scrutiny, the profession will need to look carefully at itself and ensure that, from both a public and a professional point of view, all steps are taken to assure quality, and that 'self' regulation means just that. Clinical governance is part of this. Unless the profession takes care of its own problems, others will do it.

8. **Co-operation among specialties**

With increasing specialization, there has been a tendency recently for the profession to speak with different voices, and to appear fragmented. Perhaps the time has come to be more integrated and collegiate.

What action is required now?

What we need is a full debate on the purpose of medicine and its basic values; a continuing review of medical education—in a time of change this is a key issue; an examination of standards and quality in clinical practice; further consideration of the organization of medicine—looking to the year 2000 and beyond; and a recognition of the responsibility of the profession to take these forward.

3. The future of specialization in medicine

Introduction

The subject of specialization in medicine is an important one and is relevant to all countries and health care systems. Throughout the world health care administrations are struggling with the problem and how to deal with it; in particular, the issues surrounding education and training, manpower and staffing, financial considerations, and how best to deliver the service within finite resources. Above all, how to do this whilst still meeting public and patient expectations of high-quality services. This section will cover some, but not all of the issues, and the examples used will be mainly from the UK.

Two final introductory points: first, that the transference of any aspect of the health system of one country, to another, is rarely successful and is not advocated here; second, that the care for the patient and for the community is paramount, and should be the focus of attention.

In one sense specialization is not new. There have been physicians and surgeons and apothecaries going back to medieval times. In the last 20 to 30 years however there has been an explosion in the number of specialties which have been developed and recognized by various medical bodies and professional associations. Within my own lifetime the specialties of oncology, clinical genetics, clinical pharmacology, paediatric nephrology and intensive care medicine have all developed. Even specialties which may seem to be well established, such as orthopaedics, have a relatively short history. The trend is undoubtedly for more specialization rather than less. It is the consequences of this which will be examined here. The context within which this is occurring also needs to be considered. The way in which health care is delivered is changing rapidly, with advances in medicine, and changes in the demographic pattern of the population. Public expectations are now higher than ever that the quality of care delivered will be of the highest order, and that such health care will be available to them no matter where they live. The development of specialist practice must also be placed within the context of the continuum of medical education of which it is only one part. The consequences of developing specialist practice, its affordability, and its link to financial and human resources also needs to be considered. Specialization may not be the only way forward: the role of the generalist also needs to be considered.

The characteristics of a specialist

This section attempts to analyse the characteristics of professional practice and to outline the kind of doctor who is required in any society. This will vary very considerably depending on the availability of doctors and other health professionals, and also on public expectations, and will be determined by the kind of health care system established by the political process.

What then do we mean by a specialist? The cynic might describe the specialist as someone who knows more and more about less and less. However, over the last year or so, as thinking has developed, the characteristics of a specialist have been more clearly defined to include someone who has a particular interest in the clinical area, and who has made a special study of it, has undertaken further education and training, and has an extended knowledge base. In addition, the individual has a link to other specialists. There is a temptation to use the term specialist in a very narrow way. However, this would be too restrictive because, for example, the general practitioner is a specialist in family medicine and a general physician, in general internal medicine. 'Supra' specialists, in whatever clinical area, are thus not the only ones for to whom the term can be used.

One of the most important aspects of the discussion is the relationship between the specialist doctor and the specialist service. While an individual doctor may be trained to specialist level, it would be very difficult for her or him to practice without contact with other specialist doctors or professional groups, such as nurses, who have their own particular specialist skills. A key part of being a specialist, therefore, is of working within a team of clinical staff, all of whom are working towards the same objective of better patient care. A few examples of necessary close collaboration will illustrate this more appropriately:

1. In the management of breast cancer, a medical oncologist must collaborate with a radiotherapist, surgeon, pathologist, specialist nurses, and so on.

2. Those concerned with ENT practice collaborate with plastic surgeons, dental surgeons, speech therapists, and so on.
3. In orthopaedics, the surgeon collaborates with biomedical engineers and physiotherapists.
4. In diabetes, the physician collaborates with chiropodists, dieticians, ophthalmologists, and so on.

Thus being a specialist, without a link to a specialist service and a role within multidisciplinary and multiprofessional teams, is likely to be insufficient.

Evidence for the value of specialization

One of the key questions which is asked by decision makers is whether specialization actually improves patient care. It is surprisingly difficult to identify such evidence. In cancer care, a recent paper by Selby, Gillis, and Haward (1996) reviewed the evidence currently available.[3] They concluded that it was fairly strong in some cancers—notably breast cancer, ovarian cancer, some haematological malignancies, and some childhood cancers—but beyond that, the evidence was lacking. The key features which were identified were the importance of training, the case-load, and working within multidisciplinary teams. Improved outcomes could be achieved within a network of district general hospitals which were linked to specialist centres. A second piece of evidence published in a recent *Effective Healthcare Bulletin* (1996) summarized the relationship between volume and outcome in clinical practice.[4] The conclusions were that the data was of mixed quality and that there was no general relationship between the two. However, in some specialties it could be demonstrated that there was good evidence that specialization did result in better outcomes. There is clearly very much more work to be done in relation to effectiveness and outcomes, and in defining the quality of care. One of the major functions of specialist medical bodies such as colleges and academies should be to develop this evidence. Quality of care is a very important value for a professional group.

The training of specialists

In considering the future of specialization it is inevitable that the issue of the training of specialists needs particular discussion. Recently in the UK the model of specialist training has been revised (The Calman Report, 1993)[5], in response to pressure from the European Commission. The revised model builds on existing processes, with the only one new component being that the end point assessment is based on the competence of the doctor on completion of specialist training. Entry into the training grade, now known as the Specialist Registrar Grade, is competitive, as before. The Registrar and Senior Registrar grades have been combined, and during the process of training—which itself is structured and planned—there is increased supervision and a regular review of progress. The curriculum, including the minimum length of time in which training should be completed, is devised by the specialist medical groups, generally the Medical Royal Colleges. The end assessment is based on competency, and the individual is awarded a Certificate of Completion of Specialist Training (CCST). As already stated, this is the only new part of the process. A new Specialist Training Authority (STA) has been set up, and once an individual has been given the CCST he or she is registered with the General Medical Council (GMC) in a specialist register. By April 1997, 13 000 trainees in 52 specialties had begun the new process of training. This has been the easy part; the difficult part will be ensuring the quality of the educational process and in the assessment of competency. Before an individual can become a consultant in the National Health Service in the UK, he or she is required to be registered as a specialist by the GMC.

With the bulk of the training programmes up and running, three areas require further consideration. These have already been the subject of Working Party Reports but, as the process itself unfolds, they will need further refining. The first area relates to those individuals in academic and research posts. British medicine has always had a strong academic and research tradition and it is important that in the process of change, the flexibility and the encouragement to enter academic and research medicine is not limited in any way. Special mechanisms have been introduced to ensure that this continues, but further discussion is required. The second area is that of general practice. The consequences of the new training programme on general practice continues to be thought through, and the process of education in general practice itself is changing. More work is required in this area. The third area concerns overseas doctors who come to the UK for further specialist training. In 1997, the Home Office changed its rules for postgraduate education and training, and it is now possible for those from overseas to come to the UK for a period of training which is not time limited, as long as the individual is part of a postgraduate training programme and that progress is satisfactory. Individuals from overseas can come as before and carry out periods of short- or long-term training, and those who wish full specialist training can enter programmes which will lead to the award of an equivalent of a CCST. The contribution that overseas doctors make to training and service in the UK is very considerable and these new changes should not restrict entry.

More and more people in specialist practice wish their training to be done flexibly and on a part-time basis. This is to be encouraged and mechanisms are in place for ensuring greater flexibility in training, over a longer period of time, whilst allowing the individual to complete training to an appropriate level.

Continuing professional development

One of the most important aspects of being a consultant or specialist is the need to keep up to date. The quality of care needs to continue to be of the highest level, and this can be assured in a variety of ways including mentoring, peer review, and continuing medical education (CME). In the UK we are moving further away from CME to continuing professional development (CPD). This covers a broader range of issues than simply medical education and would include, for example, the development of management skills. CPD is an area which is of considerable importance and requires further development.

The organization of a specialist service

In England and Wales over the last few years we have been developing a model for specialist services in the cancer area (Calman/Hine Report, 1995).[6] This can serve as methodology from which general lessons can be identified and related to other conditions or groups of patients. This model focuses on patients, and is based on evidence of outcome. It is in three parts, the first being the role of the general practitioner and the primary care team, the second that of district general hospital cancer units, and the third, the development of cancer centres. The primary care team, for example, has responsibilities in relation to diagnosis, some screening procedures, some treatment, follow-up, and palliative care. The team requires guidelines for referral to the cancer unit. The cancer unit itself, based in a district general hospital, will generally treat the common cancers and will group together those clinicians in that hospital with a special interest in cancer treatment, including nurses, dieticians, and speech therapists. Once again, there is a close link between the cancer unit and the primary care team on the one hand, and the cancer unit and the specialist centre on the other. The cancer centre will generally treat most types of cancer and offer the full range of diagnostic and therapeutic facilities. It is likely to take a special interest in paediatric and adolescent disease, and to have a particular role in teaching and education and in the development of protocols and guidelines for care.

The consequences of this model are that the patient should be seen in a much more holistic way, and that the service is delivered seamlessly across the three components. There is greater public involvement and teamworking, with an integration of the care management package using guidelines which are continually evaluated and updated. However, there are also some downsides to the development of specialist services. To make the process work effectively requires adequate staffing and effective education and training arrangements. There is also the problem, which will be discussed later, of having too many specialists, and too few people to deal with patients who present with acute illness. This model of cancer services is now being used in the development of other fields of clinical work.

The disadvantages of specialization

So far in this chapter the case has been made for specialization, and for clinical care to be delivered by consultants and others who have special knowledge and training. However, there are considerable disadvantages in developing a specialist-based service. The first has already been mentioned and is in dealing with clinical emergencies. Patients do not present in neatly packaged forms, and those who deal with emergency care have to be sufficiently flexible and trained generally to deal with such conditions. The second area is in the staffing of the service. While, as has been discussed, there are benefits to specialist care, if the service is to be staffed only by specialists then most health care systems in the world would not be able to comply, either because of manpower constraints, or funding problems. The third area is perhaps the most important. British medicine has always been characterized by the general physician or general surgeon. Such individuals—'the wise physicians'—have provided, through their considerable experience, a great service to patients and the public. They are able to take a broad view of a clinical problem, ensuring that the diagnostic process is not restricted. The generalist is therefore someone to be valued, and not set aside in the process of specialization. This is not an issue of funding; it is an issue of quality of care. We lose the generalist at our peril, and to the disadvantage of patients.

The evaluation of specialist services

In the process of change in the development of specialists it is important that the service at each step is evaluated. It is also relevant to ask the question for whose benefit these changes are introduced. Are they for the patient, the public, professionals, or politicians? Changing the ways in which services are organized can be expensive, time consuming and very challenging. It is incumbent therefore on those who introduce such changes to ensure that they are properly evaluated.

The role of the public

The end point of the process, as discussed at the beginning of this chapter, is to improve the care of patients and to meet public expectations. For that reason it is important that the public are involved in the process of the development of specialist services and that their expectations are able to be debated and considered. The public have a very significant role in determining what services are provided, and patients themselves are clearly very concerned about the quality of care provided.

Some other issues

1. **Specialization of other professional groups**
It is not only in medicine that specialization is occurring. Other groups such as dieticians, nurses, pharmacists, and physiotherapists are all similarly involved in the process. This too will have consequences on clinical practice. Doctors must therefore continue to work very closely with all other professional groups in the delivery of patient care.
2. **Specialization in research**
One of the strengths of British medicine has been that many of those involved in clinical practice have had an active interest in research. It is important that this continues and that leading-edge medicine continues to be practised.

3. **Specialization in education**
As the quality of training programmes for specialists improves, a group of doctors with a specific interest in education is likely to emerge. This is an undervalued area of medicine, and one which could easily be developed further with the interest of such a group. For that reason, those with a special interest in education should be regarded the same as those who specialize in clinical practice or research. Teaching the teachers or training the trainers is a very important element of medical practice.
4. **Career advice to young doctors**
The whole of this discussion can be focused into this one area. What advice would you give to a young doctor who asks about specialist practice and the opportunities available? The answer will depend on many factors, but perhaps clarifies personal thinking in this area

Some conclusions

In this section the advantages and disadvantages of specialization have been considered. In some areas there are clear advantages in specialist practice, but there are some important disadvantages. There remains an important role for the generalist in clinical practice. The most important aspect of all is the outcome for the patient, and this should remain at the heart of medical education and the role of the doctor.

4. Do we need a new Hippocratic Oath?

Hippocrates is often regarded as the ideal physician and a role model for medical practice through the centuries. His oath has a central place in medical practice. In his teaching he emphasized the importance of diagnosis, prognosis and treatment, the role of preventive medicine, the central place of education, and the importance of ethics. To understand the Hippocratic Oath, and in particular to consider if there is a need for a new one, it is necessary to be aware of the background and to acknowledge that it was written in a particular context, that the content related to other writings, and that the concept of taking an 'oath' was also important. These three facets will now be reviewed before considering the possibility of a new 'oath'.

The context Medicine in Greece in the fourth century BC had considerable limitations in knowledge, technology, and therapeutic skills. However certain basic principles were established, including the importance of correctly establishing the diagnosis and assessing the prognosis. It was also made clear that treatment had not only to be effective, but should not harm the patient. The role of prevention was stressed as was the need to maintain a good diet and to take regular exercise. Particular reference was made to the importance of epidemiology and to an understanding of individuals, where they lived, and what their job was. The detailed case histories in the Hippocratic writings present a fascinating insight into the practice of medicine at the time and the need to keep detailed records of consultations. The *Aphorisms* are also an important source of information on medical practice and offer practical comments on a wide range of clinical issues. The scientific method was just developing; the knowledge base was naturally very small.

The content The Hippocratic Oath is a very practical document, full of good clinical advice, though it is often considered to be only concerned with ethical issues and a pronouncement on moral principles. While this is undoubtedly true, it is more than this, and includes statements on teaching, treatment, and professional standards. For this reason, if the oath is to be reviewed it requires more therefore than an updated statement of ethical issues. It needs to be a working document for the practising doctor—as was the original oath.

The concept Oaths are perhaps now a little out of fashion, and the modern equivalent would be a promise, a pledge, or a declaration. It is still seen as part of professional ethics to take a pledge, or make a promise about professional standards. A number of medical schools still administer an oath before graduation. In this context an 'oath' is a personal statement or promise, as opposed to a 'charter' which confers rights and privileges on others.

The current Hippocratic Oath

The actual oath of Hippocrates is given here for reference:

I swear by Apollo the physician, and Aesculapius, and Health, and All-heal, and all the gods and goddesses, that, according to my ability and judgement, I will keep this Oath and this stipulation—to reckon him who taught me this Art equally dear to me as my parents, to share my substance with him, and relieve his necessities if required; to look upon his offspring on the same footing as my own brothers, and to teach them this art, if they shall wish to learn it, without fee or stipulation; and that by precept, lecture, and every other mode of instruction, I will impart a knowledge of the Art to my own sons, and those of my teachers, but to none others. I will follow that system or regimen which, according to my ability and judgement, I consider for the benefit of my patients, and abstain from whatever is deleterious and mischievous. I will give no deadly medicine to any one if asked, nor suggest any such counsel; and in like manner I will not give to a woman a pessary to produce abortion. With purity and with holiness I will pass my life and practise my Art. I will not cut persons labouring under the stone, but will leave this to be done by men who are practitioners of this work.

Into whatever houses I enter, I will go into them for the benefit of the sick, and will abstain from every voluntary act of mischief and corruption; and, further, from the seduction of females or males, of freemen and slaves. Whatever, in connection with my professional practice or not in connection with it, I see or hear in the life of men, which ought not to be spoken of abroad, I will not divulge, as reckoning that all such should be kept secret. While I continue to keep this Oath unviolated, may it be granted to me to enjoy life and the practice of the Art, respected by all men, in all times! But should I trespass and violate this Oath, may the reverse be my lot!

The need for a review

With greater public awareness about medical issues and the ways in which doctors work, there is increasing public concern about medical practice and professional standards. There is less respect for doctors, and the variations in practice and results which are noted, emphasize possible differences in effectiveness and, thus, inequalities in the care provided. It is for this reason that a restatement is perhaps necessary. This very personal reinterpretation is offered as a contribution to the debate on the future role of the doctor. The 'Promise' is presented as a series of statements based on the Hippocratic Oath, each of which is followed by an explanation or development of the theme.

The new 'promise' **I promise as part of the wider Fellowship of the medical profession, to uphold the long-established traditions of care, compassion, commitment, and service, and to maintain and improve standards of health and health care given to individual patients and the community.**
This introduction to the 'promise' recognizes the international fellowship of medicine and its long traditions. It also, indirectly, indicates that the doctor has a role as a citizen, as well as a professional. The responsibilities extended beyond the individual patient to the community and the population as a whole. It emphasizes that the purpose of medical practice is to serve the patient and the public. Thus, the public health role and the importance of social and economic factors in health and illness are noted.

1. I will put the quality of life and the health of patients and the community I serve first, and act as an advocate on their behalf.
This establishes the prime function of the doctor and stresses the importance of health as well as illness. Quality of life is seen as crucial. The doctor has a vital role, in association with others, as an advocate for the patient. It also identifies one of the crucial tensions—care for the patient versus responsibility for the community.
2. In my relationships with patients and the public I will recognize the importance of communication,

and of involving them in choices and making decisions.
Communication is central to medical practice, whether it be with the patient, the family or friends, or the public. It is a two-way process, and involves listening and explaining. Patient involvement and participation is essential to promote trust and ensure that the patient is part of the process of care. For those with a special interest in public health, this need for involvement of the community is equally important.

3. I will respect the dignity of individual patients and be sensitive to their personal beliefs. I will treat all equally. I will maintain strict confidentiality of all information divulged to me by patients. I will preserve the values and ethical principles of the medical profession.
The ethical basis of medical practice is defined in this section. Part of this is the need to treat all, equally, regardless of race, colour, creed, or personal lifestyle. Confidentiality of the information disclosed in the relationship is also seen to be relevant to current medical practice. It is a further factor in the establishment of trust. Values are the basis of ethical principles.

4. I will practise my art to the highest standards of quality and excellence. I will continually evaluate the quality of my work.
This recognizes the educational basis of medical practice and the need to set and maintain standards of excellence. This must involve self-learning and an acknowledgement of the importance of continuing medical education. The process of setting standards and auditing the quality of work, together with the need to continually improve the quality of personal performance, are very much part of this. The measurement of the outcomes of medical care is central.

5. I will practise my art with humility, recognizing my own limitations and the skills of others. I will work within the team context.
Arrogance is a common failing of the medical profession; humility would be more appropriate. It is essential to work

to deliver health care or public health measures within a team context, and to acknowledge the skills of other members of the team. Much of clinical work is problem solving, and this provides the opportunity to work and learn together. Interprofessional education is thus relevant at all stages of professional development.

6. I will recognize that the decisions I make will have consequences for the patient, the community, and for resources.

The diagnosis is a key element in making decisions. There are a range of dimensions associated with making a diagnosis, and the consequences in terms of prognosis and treatment are crucial. The consultation and subsequent diagnosis are the building blocks of health care. It is the diagnosis which establishes requirements in terms of resources (which, in this context, include time, skills and expertise, facilities, and funding).

7. I will not consciously harm the individual or community I care for; nor will I take advantage of or use in any way, my special relationship with them.

This is an important issue. In general terms it is about non-malevolence, and the need to ensure that patients are fully involved in the decision-making process. At a deeper level, it is also about not abusing the special relationship and trust between the patient and the doctor, for example, in relation to commercial interests. Further, it can relate to even more sinister issues including torture of a physical or psychological nature.

8. I will see teaching and the transmission of my experience to others as part of my role as a doctor.

This emphasizes the importance of teaching for the doctor. (Indeed the derivation of the word 'doctor' indicates its roots in teaching.) This oath also draws out the responsibilities doctors have to each other, to pass on knowledge, skills, and attitudes. In this context the hidden curriculum in medicine is relevant. There is, for example, the moral responsibility to keep up to date, thus ensuring that to the best of one's ability, patients get the most relevant and appropriate advice.

9. I will base my practice on the twin principles of scientific observation and enquiry, and a humanitarian and holistic approach.
It is clear that medical practice needs to be embedded in the scientific method and to be knowledge based. On the other hand there is a requirement for an holistic and humanitarian approach. Both breadth and depth are required of the doctor. At different periods of education and in different phases of one's career, these will have different emphases.
10. I will see it as part of my duty to improve health and health care by research and development.
The curiosity motive is strong in those engaged in clinical and public health practice. There is a great need for research to push back the frontiers of knowledge and, in so doing, improve health and health care. A greater awareness of what determines health and the outcome of health care will be the main way in which improvements can occur. All doctors should have this curiosity motive. But there is, of course, more to it than this. It is also about the implementation of research findings and of ensuring that new knowledge is fully used. In this respect doctors should be agents of change and, as major opinion formers, should be leading the move for change.
11. While my commitment to clinical practice will be full, I will ensure that my life is balanced with outside interests, and will give time to family and friends.
I will maintain a sense of proportion, purpose, and humour. To do this I will try to develop:
- confidence—without arrogance
- courtesy and respect for the feelings and the rights of others
- competence—but a willingness to still learn
- commitment to caring and professional standards, and to outside interests and family and friends
- contentment with medical life; fulfilment and satisfaction with outside interests.

A summary of the new promise I promise as part of the wider Fellowship of the medical profession, to uphold the long-established traditions of care, compassion, commitment, and service, and to maintain and improve standards of health and health care given to individual patients and the community.

1. I will put the quality of life and the health of patients and the community I serve first, and act as an advocate on their behalf.
2. In my relationships with patients and the public, I will recognize the importance of communication, and of involving them in choices and making decisions.
3. I will respect the dignity of individual patients and be sensitive to their personal beliefs. I will treat all equally. I will maintain strict confidentiality of all information divulged to me by patients. I will preserve the values and ethical principles of the medical profession.
4. I will practise my art to the highest standards of quality and excellence. I will continually evaluate the quality of my work.
5. I will practise my art with humility, recognizing my own limitations and the skills of others. I will work within the team context.
6. I will recognize that the decisions I make will have consequences for the patient, the community, and resources.
7. I will not consciously harm the individual or community I care for; nor will I take advantage of, or use in any way, my special relationship with them.
8. I will see teaching and the transmission of my experience to others as part of my role as a doctor.
9. I will base my practice on the twin principles of scientific observation and enquiry, and a humanitarian and holistic approach.
10. I will see it as part of my duty to improve health and health care by research and development.
11. While my commitment to clinical practice will be full, I will ensure that my life is balanced with outside interests, giving time to family and friends.

5. Professional education

***'A properly planned and carefully conducted medical education remains the foundation of a comprehensive Health Service.'* Goodenough, 1944**

This section covers a range of issues related to professional education. Medical education is used as the model, but the principles are relevant to other groups. The quotation at the start of this section sets the tone. Professional education is the foundation for the health service, and at the same time, the key to change. Two issues are relevant here to professional education: first, that values are important in education; and second, that one of the purposes of education is to transmit such values, as well as facts and information.

What sort of doctor?

It is impossible nowadays to go to a medical meeting, particularly one related to education, without this question being raised. Several models or, more correctly, caricatures, are available. In Richard Gordon's books we have Sir Lancelot Sprat—autocratic, distinguished, effective (but soft hearted)—and Simon Sparrow—uncertain but caring. Sir Luke Filde's picture of the physician is of someone caring, concerned, and close to the patient. Dr Finlay and Dr Cameron, as portrayed by A. J. Cronin, provide two views of general practice: the older, irascible but well-liked; the younger, aggressive and keen to change. Bernard Shaw's portrait of the research physician in *The doctor's dilemma* can be replicated in many different places. The media, notably television, provide the public and the profession with many different role models, in medicine, nursing, and other professions.

Putting all of this together, it seems that we need a 'super' doctor (female or male) who has some, or all, of the following:

- care and compassion
- encyclopaedic knowledge

- high level of technical skill
- interest in research
- ability to be a team player, a prima donna, and a citizen.

It is clearly impossible to find all this in a single person. But what it does argue for is a medical curriculum which is sufficiently flexible to allow for different end points and a range of doctors, not just a single model. What is clear, however, is that medical students and those in training are subject to a hidden agenda of values as they watch and observe their seniors in practice. Role modelling by students should not be underestimated.

The purpose of medical education

Although it is difficult to be precise about the kind of doctor required, it should be possible to set out the purpose of medical education. The following definition may be helpful:

> The purpose of medical education is to produce a doctor who will provide a high-quality service to the individual and the community; who will continue to learn and develop professionally throughout his or her professional career; who will assess professional performance regularly; and who will seek to continually improve the service provided, by research and development, within the context of the team approach.

This definition highlights a number of needs, some of which have already been raised, but will be noted here together for convenience:

(1) for the end point of medical education to be the development of a doctor who can provide a high-quality service to patients and the community;
(2) to have both an individual and community focus;
(3) for the doctor, at all stages of his or her career, to have 'lifelong' learning as part of their ethos and culture;
(4) to audit performance and continually improve outcomes;
(5) to be willing to change the boundaries of their profession and specialty;
(6) to be part of a team in the delivery of care; the patient of course also being part of the team.

Increasingly there is a wish for the public (represented in a number of ways) to be involved in determining the kind of doctor required, and influencing the process and content of the curriculum. A variety of ways have already been found to ensure this (by lay membership of the GMC, for example) but others are required.

The process of medical education

Medical education can be considered to be in three parts, each linked by the thread of lifelong learning. The first is in the medical school and university, and is generally called undergraduate or basic medical education. It lasts for five years, with a further year in hospital practice before the young doctor becomes fully registered as a medical practitioner by the GMC. It is the GMC which has overall responsibility for the supervision of all stages of medical education, together with the Special Training Authority (STA), a new body which deals with specialist education, and the Joint Committee for Training in General Practice. The second phase is that of postgraduate medical education, lasting around seven to ten years, during which increasing skills are acquired and the doctor specializes, either in general practice, public health, or one of the hospital specialties. Finally there is the period of continuing education, or continuing professional development, which lasts for the remainder of the doctor's career. This continuity is of vital importance and it is not possible to consider any of these phases in isolation. Having said that, each phase, together with relevant issues, will now be considered in more detail.

The undergraduate phase This takes place in the universities, medical schools, hospitals, and community. It is, in one sense, a remarkable process. An 18-year-old young woman or man, generally straight from school, is transformed over a period of five years into someone who can make a diagnosis, assess outcome, outline treatment (and administer it in some cases), carry out a series of clinical procedures, and communicate with patients about highly complex, difficult, and life-threatening problems. The calibre of student is very high, and they are greatly motivated to do well, and are committed to looking after patients. If they fail, it is most likely that the system has failed. Those in authority and who have responsibility for medical education must not let down these remarkable people.

The undergraduate course, in all countries, is undergoing change and revision, and the UK is no exception. The publication *Tomorrow's doctors* and the *New Doctor*, by the GMC, has set the pattern of a core curriculum; more student-centred learning; an emphasis on public health, ethics, and communication skills; the setting of clear objectives; and more relevant examination systems. The options are wide and varied, and there are generally opportunities for the student during an 'elective' period to go to another part of the country, or abroad. The current changes in the undergraduate curriculum promise an improved quality of graduate.

At the end of this process the young doctor spends a year in clinical practice (generally in two six-month periods) and is then finally fully registered with the GMC if progress has been satisfactory. The registration process is for the public good, and allows the citizen to identify fully qualified doctors from a list, or register, maintained by the GMC. This is an important measure of quality assurance.

Women in medicine There is an increasing number of women entering medical school. In some universities, over 50 per cent of students are female. This is to be welcomed, as one of the themes in this book is the important role of women in health and health care. This increase in female entrants at the undergraduate level is not, however, reflected in all specialties at the most senior levels. There are a number of reasons for this, but it is to be expected that, over time, and with encouragement, the percentage of women in senior posts will increase.

Postgraduate education Following the university training and house officer posts, the young graduate spends a variable period (one to three years) in a variety of specialty positions before proceeding to specialist training. In general practice, this includes supervised training in the practice setting. As already described, specialist education is undergoing a major transformation in the UK which will result in a more structured training period (generally shorter than before) that ends in an assessment of competence and the award of a Certificate of Completion of Specialist Training (CCST) by the Special Training Authority (STA), with subsequent placement on the specialist register of the GMC. The public will have access to this information. The Medical Royal Colleges will be involved in the assessment of competence and the setting of standards, and the Postgraduate Deans will have responsibility for managing the process at regional level.

The link between education and manpower One of the topics which has been discussed in detail over the years is how to get the numbers right—starting from intake to medical school and ending up with the right number of qualified specialists, general practitioners, and public health doctors. In general the system has worked well, though inevitably there has been surpluses and deficits. No other country seems to have achieved the 'holy grail', and most look to the UK with envy. However, things could be improved and new mechanisms have recently been set up to make this happen.

Continuing medical education (CME); continuing professional development (CPD) This is perhaps the most important, but least developed part of medical education. Good doctors have always kept up to date, reviewed their practice, and continually improved it. But the pace of change at present in medical care is so great, that this cannot be left to chance and needs to be embedded in clinical practice. It must be practice-based, problem-related, and associated with the individual's needs. The philosophy of 'lifelong, self-directed' learning must start in the medical school, or before that, to ensure that it is part of the practice and culture of every doctor.

The term CME could be considered to focus narrowly on medical education only, and for that reason the broader term CPD is increasingly used. This includes not only CME, but education in management, economics, sociology, and so on, and also personal development. It emphasizes that as people and jobs change, each doctor has to think about the way in which they develop and achieve their own potential. The vast majority of doctors work very hard for the health service. However, if they are appointed as consultants and principals in general practice in their late 20s or early 30s, then they will face 30 or more years in the same job. It is for this reason that they may need to find ways of refreshing their clinical practice, accepting new challenges, and finding increasingly fulfilling roles. CME and CPD are perhaps the most exciting areas of professional education at the present time. If solutions can be found not only will we have a workforce which is continually improving its practice and is actively seeking new ways forward, but patient care will also improve.

Some educational issues

The process of medical education has been described first in order to allow a discussion of educational issues to be set in context. These can now be considered in more detail.

Education and training It is proper to make a distinction between the two terms, though in practice they overlap. Training is generally considered to be directed to the acquisition of specific knowledge or skills. Education is broader and, in addition, is also concerned with values. This is why a university education, in which medical students rub shoulders with students from other faculties and disciplines, is considered to be important. In shorthand, 'to be trained is to have arrived, to be educated is to continue to travel'. Or to use a mapping analogy, training is concerned with the detail of some aspects of the map, education with the map as a whole.

In general we need educated doctors who are capable of meeting new challenges and seeing new possibilities and connections. Of course they need to be trained and skilled in diagnosis and treatment. But they also need to be human beings who can relate to others and show empathy and compassion. The educational philosopher R. S. Peters wrote that the highest point of education was the ability to converse on a variety of subjects, with a range of people. This ability to communicate is a fundamental part of being a doctor and this is discussed in detail elsewhere (see Chapter 10). Doctors also need to have breadth and depth, and interests outside medicine. They need to be with people who have experience of life and its emotional ups and downs. In the mid 1980s, with Professor Downie, Professor of Moral Philosophy at the University of Glasgow, a series of seminars on literature and medicines was set up. Books, plays, poems were covered, and the course has now expanded to take on a wider range of arts and the humanities. The purpose was to encourage students to think beyond the medical texts and to experience insights into the great writers and thinkers. The seminars were well-received and provided a window on to the wider world. This is described further in Chapter 6.

The concept of the curriculum Every medical school, at one point or another, has faced the problem of changing or modifying its curriculum. Around the country some very exciting developments are taking place including community-based medical schools, problem-based education, self-directed learning, and integrated learning with other professional groups. Clearer objectives are being set and better assessment of outcomes carried out.

One of the problems, however, is that the concept of the curriculum, while being applied at the undergraduate level, is less used in postgraduate and continuing education programmes. The curriculum comprises four parts. First, the aims and objectives, set out in a form which shows the learner the direction of travel and what he or she is expected to be able to do at the end of a period of study. 'Give the student a copy of the objectives and you may not need to do much more' is a well-known educational phrase. A statement of the content, the range of subjects, and their connection to other disciplines or bodies of knowledge then follows. This is the 'syllabus' and is generally the part of the curriculum which is readily available to the student. Thirdly, there is the teaching method to be used—lecture, small-group teaching, computer-based, self-directed, and so on. This is a crucial choice and sets the tone for the learning experience. Much of this is available for undergraduate courses and, to a lesser extent, for the other stages of education. Where it is not available it needs to be implemented with some urgency.

Finally, having set the curriculum, the next stage is to assess performance using appropriate methods, and this aspect will now be considered.

Assessment of competence The objective of any educational process is to change behaviour in order that new skills or knowledge be acquired, or existing ones improved. To measure the effectiveness of the process is the aim of assessment. This is one of the most difficult parts of the whole educational process, and considerable effort has gone into devising better validated methods which actually measure competence and performance. These range from written examinations, observation of clinical skills, multiple choices, objective structured clinical examinations (OSCE), peer review, self-assessment, and many others. Yet this is the area that the public are particularly concerned about—the quality of medical care provided, and the assurance that those who practice have the right skills and knowledge.

The assessment of competence is not a new problem; consider Aristotle in Book III of *Politics*. There he says:

> First, the proper person to judge whether a piece of medical work has been properly done is the same sort of person as is actually engaged on such work, on curing the patient of his present sickness—in other words the medical practitioner himself. And this is equally true of the other skills and empirical crafts. As then it is amongst doctors that a doctor should give account of himself, so also should other professional men among their peers.

And, most recently, from the *Journal of the History of Medicine*, in an article with the unusual title 'The function of praise in the contract of a medieval public physician', which looks at the history of contracts between the civil authorities and doctors, drawing on Greek and Roman experience:

Roman policy makers faced the same basic problems that the Greeks had encountered before them. How could they develop a meaningful mechanism to evaluate the proficiency of a member of a profession that possessed a specialised knowledge beyond the ken of the uninitiated? Or, to put more simply how could lawyers recognise expertise outside their own province? It was an important question because some workable system was necessary to guarantee the quality of public services.

The Romans found, as the Greeks had, that the most practical way to discover whether or not an applicant was qualified for a civic position, was by the hazy criterion of public renown. In the absence of any professional licensing body, the Romans had to rely on the good reputation of the physician and to determine this they utilised the testimony of teachers, friends, and grateful cities as well as public contests . . . and to choose men to whom they must entrust themselves and their children when ill.

Our patients still trust us, and they are our greatest allies.

Educational research Fundamental to all of this is the need for more research on educational issues. Some of this will be quite basic—How do we learn? What are the psychological methods involved? Can the conditions of learning be more clearly defined? Some will be of a more applied nature, dealing with a comparison of educational methods or assessment procedures. In general, educational research has not had the kind of priority that other aspects of biomedical research have enjoyed. Its status is lower, and it has been regarded, along with teaching, as of lesser importance than clinical skills and expertise. We badly need more educational research to expand and improve the quality of the educational experience.

The role of the teacher This is perhaps best summed up in the caption to a Snoopy cartoon, 'was I judged on what I learnt about this project, if so then were not you, my teacher, also being judged on your ability to transmit your knowledge to me? Are you willing to share my C?' The derivation of the word doctor comes from the Latin *docere*, to teach, and one of the important roles of the doctor, from the time of Hippocrates, has been that of the teacher. But how well prepared are doctors for this function? How much time have they spent learning to teach? Teaching the teachers is one of the neglected aspects of medical education. It is assumed that a highly qualified doctor will naturally have an innate ability to teach and, while some have, others could improve. Teachers, of course, should not be considered as the person who stands up and passes on wisdom and knowledge, but as someone who facilitates the learning of the student. As a 'learning problem solver' the teacher, with the student, identifies learning needs and selects the appropriate method to use. Teaching is therefore about choosing the right learning experiences for the learner. There is a clear need to recognize the value of teaching and the role of the teacher as a leader.

The role of the learner As has been said repeatedly, each individual doctor has a responsibility to learn throughout his or her career. Everyone learns rather differently, and if the question is asked 'How do doctors learn?', then there are several answers. Inevitably books and journals form part of the process, as does attendance at meetings, conferences, and lectures. These however are relatively inefficient methods and it is suggested (with less evidence than I would like) that most practical learning is by face to face contact with a colleague about a particular patient-related problem. If the question is asked, 'What did I learn that changed my practice recently?', then the answer is likely to be related to a clinical problem, the discussion of which, with colleagues and senior members, provides a forum, not only to 'hear the expert', but also to exchange views and share problems. Much more work is needed on improving the learning environment.

Communication skills

This topic has been raised throughout this book, and several times in this chapter. It is a key skill, requiring practice and refinement, and the component of medical practice which impinges most on the patient. Almost all medical schools have recognized this, and it should be part of the assessment for postgraduate and continuing education.

Ethical implications
In addition to practising medicine according to clear ethical principles, doctors also have an obligation to keep up to date. It is not in the interests of patient care to be seen by a doctor whose skills and knowledge base are 20 years behind the times. For all doctors to be right at the leading edge of their specialty is unrealistic and, in some instances, not necessary. Many new techniques may not have been assessed and may turn out to be of limited value. But they do all have an obligation to ensure that they practice to the best of their ability and review their performance regularly. This is the clear educational link to audit (see Chapter 10) and the use of standards and guidelines for treatment.

Specialist or generalist? One of the most interesting debates in medicine (and other professions) at the present time is that of the balance between the generalist and the specialist. On the one hand the greater the expertise and skill of the practitioner, the better for the patient with a specific illness or disease. On the other hand there is the danger of overdiagnosis or underdiagnosis if a general view is not taken. For many medical complaints a breadth of view is required, together with a high index of suspicion. The gatekeeper role of the generalist is an important one. The balance varies from country to country, and even from specialty to specialty. The educational issue is how best to plan training programmes to meet both needs and give sufficient breadth of experience. For those planning the curriculum, and those managing the process, this needs to be taken into account.

A formal component of CME For a number of years now there has been discussion on the best way to ensure that CME programmes are being taken up by individual doctors. The airline pilots' analogy is generally used. Pilots undergo a regular and planned series of performance reviews to ensure that they are up to scratch, and as a form of public assurance. If pilots can do it, why not doctors, nurses, and other health care professionals? It is for this reason that a number of educational bodies are considering mandatory reaccreditation or recertification. The introduction of the CCST, referred to earlier, could provide the reference point for each individual on which recertification would then be based. Similar systems operate in other countries.

Before embarking on this however, some quite difficult issues must be thought through. These include the methodology employed in the assessment, the measurement of the performance, and what to do if the doctor does not meet the requirements. This is the subject of the next section.

The poor doctor Most doctors perform well, are highly regarded, and, in opinion polls, regularly come out near the top in public esteem. They constitute, like other health care groups, a very committed group of professionals with a wish to serve patients and the public. The GMC has a procedure to deal with those with serious professional problems, the final sanction being removal of the doctor's name from the register and, thus, the ability to practice medicine. For doctors whose performance is consistently poor, new procedures are being introduced. However, there remains a group of doctors whose performance is poor, but not sufficiently so to remove them from the register, and it is this group which requires further consideration. The first approach is preventive—identifying at an early stage issues which might cause a problem and dealing with them. This measure is already used during undergraduate and postgraduate education, and steps are under way to improve it over the next few years. The second approach is that of clinical audit, applied as part of continuing education and development. If these two methods fail, then a third one is to introduce mandatory retraining, with performance assessment. However, if the process of CME and certification are effective, the numbers requiring this retraining will be small. Doctors, however, are human beings and can succumb to alcohol and drugs like the population as a whole. Such doctors need identification and special programmes of rehabilitation.

A particularly important group are those doctors who are professionally isolated, either by geography, or by the fact that their specialty is small and those practising it, widely dispersed. Special arrangements may be necessary to assist these doctors by some form of mentoring or peer review. Such approaches also have wider applicability for all specialists and general practitioners. Some specialties, for example, thoracic medicine, are already using mentoring and peer review on a voluntary basis, and much will be learned from this experience.

Management education Doctors and other health professionals spend a lot of their time managing patients and resources. If resources (for example, the doctor's time) are used for one purpose, they obviously cannot be used for another. But management education is broader than just looking after resources and the curriculum covers planning, strategy, personal management, budgeting, and leadership. At all stages of the medical career it should be possible to integrate management education programmes. If those responsible for the assessment of professional standards placed management issues within the context of the course, it is likely that the matter would receive the serious attention it requires. The increasing role of doctors, and other health professionals, in the management of health care marks this as an important step forward and one to be encouraged. It would be a good opportunity for interprofessional education based around case studies or problem solving.

The future

Medical education is at a very exciting stage. There is much innovation and creativity. Change is occurring more rapidly than might have been thought possible, and all is directed at improving the quality of patient care. There are some difficult issues—assessment of competence, the value of CME and CPD, and dealing with the poor doctor are just a few of them. But this activity is to be welcomed, as is the greater status given to the role of the teacher and educational research. Much is happening elsewhere in other countries which is equally exciting and breaks new ground. Such developments need to be monitored carefully and every effort taken to use them to build on what is already happening in this country. What has been described in this chapter is the beginning of a rapid evolution in education.

6. Working together: teamwork

Teamwork is not a new concept; it has always been part of good clinical practice. But it has become more important as the need to make full use of all members of the health care team has been recognized. The skill mix of the team is a matter for continuing debate, thus a discussion of this issue is particularly relevant. The purpose, as always, is to provide the highest possible quality of care to the patient and the family. Teams will only be effective if the patient-centred focus is at the heart of the process.

Teams, of course, do not replace the important therapeutic relationship between the patient and the professional. This relationship, as has been described earlier in this chapter, is crucial. Indeed the purpose of the team is to support and develop that relationship with each of the professionals involved. This will result in the patient having a sense of continuity of care from the team, and a personal sense of belonging. The values of the team—openness, commitment, compassion—are important, and are as those of the individual professional. Teams need shared aims and a shared vision.

Aims and team roles

The shared aims of the team are obviously important, but these are not spontaneously generated. They are hammered out, discussed, debated, and, by joint agreement, put into practice. This aspect is frequently missing. Within the team there are often different aims, objectives, and professional cultures, which are never brought together and systemized towards a common purpose. It is the patient who suffers if this is not done.

It should be clear that all members of the team are equal, and all are necessary. Each has a distinctive role. Effective teams require a mix of skills, and as a consequence all members of the team must recognize the skills and expertise of others. This can only happen if teams meet regularly to discuss common problems and shared goals. An analogy might help to clarify this. A football team with 11 players will be ineffective if they are all goalkeepers; a range of skills is required. The balance of skills will vary from time to time, but players need to train together, work together, discuss mistakes and failures, and build on success. So it is with clinical teams. They need to share problems and solve problems in order to develop their shared aims.

At this point, an example of a clinical team might be useful. For proper management of diabetes, for instance, the following might be required:

(1) full involvement of the patient, as without this there cannot be an effective team;
(2) a range of professionals—nurse specialists, chiropodists, social services, the voluntary sector, hospital-based doctors (diabetic physicians, ophthalmologists, vascular surgeons, and so on);
(3) primary care team that includes the general practitioner, the practice nurse, and the health visitor.

All of this needs to be managed and the outcome evaluated if the best use of this very large resource is to be obtained. In the same way the public health team will include not only public health trained doctors but nurses, environmental health officers, dentists, planners, engineers, specialists in communicable disease, and many others.

The team leader

Leadership is an important aspect of teamwork. All football teams have a captain, who may play in different positions. The captain leads, stimulates, and provides the motivation;

builds the team; and uses all the players effectively. So it is with clinical teams. We need leaders who have vision and energy, direction and purpose. But they also need knowledge, credibility, and experience. But who should be the leader of the team? Undoubtedly, the person who can do it best, and the leadership may change from time to time—it does not always have to be the centre forward. No one member of the team, in whatever professional capacity, has the right to lead the team; leadership has to be earned and won.

Developing an effective team

A vital issue in the development of teams is the measurement of their performance. This may be done through peer review of the work of the team, through clinical audit, through measurement of outcomes, and the development of standards and guidelines. These approaches raise issues of competence and the need to integrate all the professionals involved, and this is discussed further in Chapter 10 and earlier in this chapter.

A further question to be considered is the structure and shape of the team, their size, composition, and stability. While teams vary enormously in size and composition, it is their effectiveness which is most important. Teams which include junior members of staff in training are often remarkably unstable because of the rapid turnover of personnel. A common experience for juniors is to enter a new team without being aware of its culture and ethos. This can be a difficult transition and it is perhaps not surprising therefore that new members of a team are often disruptive until they understand the value base. A period of induction is therefore necessary, and is one of the responsibilities of the team leader. This difficulty is not peculiar to clinical teams; it relates to the development of all groups.

So far it has been assumed that teams are universal, but this is not always the case. A number of professionals work very much on their own, either by choice or through force of circumstances. Professional isolation is a difficult issue in clinical practice. Such individuals do need professional support for continuing professional development, and this is particularly the case for those in primary care. Links with other professionals are essential to maintain and improve competence.

It would be strange not to mention team spirit. The ethics or culture of the team is crucial, and members meeting and getting to know each other socially, as well as at work, is part of this. This social element of teamwork, having a meal together, perhaps more appropriately known as teambuilding, is essential if the process is to develop. Communication is central to team development and must be seen as part of the leadership function. It is about listening and sharing.

It is perhaps not surprising that conflict surfaces within teams, and each team must develop a mechanism for recognizing and dealing with it. Whilst working together a number of moral issues can arise which may give cause for concern. Confidentiality and research would be two of these. Confidentiality is important; having decided who is part of the team and how far its membership extends, the team must establish what the boundaries for confidentiality are that need to be maintained. Research can often be difficult in teams as individuals often have different concepts of the value of research. For some it is intrusive and gets in the way of patient care; for others it is one way of continually improving the quality of care; and for yet others it is a means to an end—the achievement of a higher degree or promotion. Opportunities have to be made for such issues to be raised and discussed openly.

Team education

One of the most interesting and exciting developments in the past few years has been the increased recognition of the value of interprofessional education. At the level of undergraduate (basic) education, team learning occurs perhaps less than it might, but at the graduate (postbasic) end there is greater scope. Learning based around a common clinical problem, audit results, new methods of treatment, or delivery of care can increase the cohesion of the team, change practice, and improve care. Learning in teams should be encouraged, but the educational methods used should be based on real clinical issues, including team leadership and management, within which the experience of all members of the team can be recognized. The related skills need to be learned, and the allocation of resources for this purpose might be of a great value. Teams need managing; it is an active process developing a team and it should not be assumed that everyone can do it without help.

The patient's role

It has been assumed, so far, that the patient is part of the team, though perhaps this should now be stated explicitly. Good two-way communication between the patient and the professional has been emphasized several times in this book already. Patient participation groups, with their increasing openness and communication between staff and patients, are to be welcomed, as are any methods of assisting with this. Without the full confidence of patients and their part in making decisions, teams will not be effective and will lack purpose. Just as importantly the relatives and friends are part of the team and should be involved in decision making. Both patients and relatives often feel confused and wonder where to go for advice, information, and support. One of the functions of the team (and of the leader) is to provide such help.

Conclusions

But are teams worthwhile? The general consensus is that they are if they provide a range of skills and experience, working to a common purpose, and that the different perspectives of the various professionals, managers, and patients are reconciled. The 'therapeutic community' which is developed is one way of achieving the aim of high-quality care. Looking ahead it is likely that the concept of the team will develop further within the context of the patient–professional relationship.

References

1. Calman, K. C. (1994). The profession of medicine. *BMJ*, **309**, 1140–43.
2. Irvine, D. (1997). The performance of doctors I: Professionalism and self regulation in a changing world. *BMJ*, **314**, 1540–42.
3. Irvine, D. (1997). The performance of doctors II: Maintaining good practice, protecting patients from poor performance. *BMJ*, **314**, 1613–15.
4. (1993). *Learning to succeed. Report of the National Commission on Education*. Heinemann, London.
5. Selby, D., Gillis, C., and Haward, R. (1996). Benefits from specialised cancer centres. *Lancet*, **348**, 313–18.
6. (1996). *Effective health care bulletin, 2, No. 8. Hospital volume and health care outcomes, costs and patient access*. Churchill Livingstone.
7. Calman, K. C. (1993). *Hospital doctors: training for the future. The report of the Working Group on Specialist Medical Training (The Calman Report)*. Department of Health.
8. Expert Advisory Group on Cancer. (1993) *A policy for commissioning cancer services*. Department of Health.

13

Looking to the future: some big issues ahead

1. Introduction

Predicting the future is difficult, and perhaps it might be better not to try. However, thinking ahead to determine possible new developments should encourage a culture of readiness for change, and an ability to react to unexpected events. Throughout this book, the emphasis on science, research, and intelligence gathering has highlighted the importance of looking ahead to the ways in which health and health care might change and improve. This chapter links readily with a previous section in the book on 'The medical detective' (see Chapter 7) which described the intelligence function.

Some of the issues in this chapter have already been raised, but they are gathered here for convenience. They may not constitute everybody's list, but that is part of the function of this book—to encourage debate and, in the jargon, assist in 'scenario planning'. The list includes many issues for further thought, representing a mixture of envisaged new developments and some current problems which remain to be resolved. They are based on thoughts in the late-1990s, and might change radically in the next few years. What is not in doubt is that health can be improved, and that research is fundamental to each of the topics raised.

2. Social and economic factors

Throughout this book the importance of social and economic factors has been emphasized. Housing, employment, homelessness, poverty are all part of this. There is no doubt about their relevance. More research is required to analyse and identify actions which can be implemented to improve health. Simplistic solutions are unlikely to bring results; local community involvement in the process is probably most effective.

1. The ageing population In all parts of the world people are living longer and, generally, with improving quality of life. However they present an enormous challenge in determining how best to care for them. Elderly people provide such wisdom and experience that they remain essential members of society with much to give. This is a social and political issue which needs broad debate and discussion. There is both a need to understand the ageing process and to improve the care given.

The actual process of ageing also requires fundamental research. The questions raised about ageing such as, do all organs age at the same rate, is there a limit to the ageing process, and can it be reversed, are basic ones which raise a host of ethical issues.

2. Disability People who are disabled have an enormous amount to give to society. Whether the disability relates to mental or physical health is immaterial. The opportunity for these people to enjoy life, and to achieve their full potential is important. Quality of life is at the heart of this and we need to encourage a culture which is both supportive and positive. In the years ahead the needs of the disabled will require to be more clearly defined, and services developed to meet such needs.

3. Quality of life This is a difficult issue to define, but it is what being healthy is about and is the end point of health care. For this reason we need better and more robust methods of measurement. Increasing the life span of the population without consideration of issues of quality of life is not necessarily the best way forward. The phrase 'compression of morbidity' has been used to describe the process by which not only is lifespan increased, but the individual experiences less disability and ill health.

4. The role of women and the family At various points in this book the importance of women and health has been signalled. Looking ahead to new issues in public health, the role of women again needs to be emphasized. So much behaviour is determined at an early stage of life, and in this the role of women remains central. The family as a unit has been under threat for some time, yet it is a great cohesive force, and a setting in which health and illness can be discussed in a supportive environment. Parenting skills may be an important issue for those who have less ready access to family and friends for support and advice.

5. *Education* People are our greatest resource, and one factor of vital importance to health is the level of education of the population—both general education and specific knowledge of health matters (health literacy). An educated population is a healthy one.

There is also a need for greater public understanding of the scientific basis of the changes in health and advances in health care, and of issues such as risk. It is the responsibility of the professionals to take part in this educational process and to encourage the public at large to feel involved.

For professional staff, education is the key to many of the changes and improvements in health and health care which lie ahead. Without a good grounding in basic education it will be increasingly difficult for doctors or any other health professionals to keep up to date and to provide high-quality care. Standards of care will become more important, encompassing the need for audit and continuing professional education and development. In addition we need to value our staff and to ensure that their welfare is always taken into account. They give a huge commitment to public service and caring for people, and we should recognize that at every opportunity.

3. Understanding disease

1. Genetic issues As the technology advances, so the implications for individual and population health will become ever clearer. For the long term, an understanding of genetic factors will probably be the most important of these. As a subset of this, advances in molecular biology will also provide new ways of looking at disease and its management. The reclassification of disease and entirely new approaches to illness will challenge conventional thinking. The human genome project will open up new avenues of research.

One of the important features of this development will be the ability to understand disease and its pathogenesis. Groups of diseases, such as coronary heart disease, could be subdivided into different categories with different prognoses and treatments. It is not just new cures we require but a fundamental understanding of why diseases occur in the first place. This emphasizes the importance of basic research work, which can often take a long time to get from the laboratory to the clinic. Without it however we will lack new ways of looking at disease and illness.

The ethical issues surrounding such advances have been discussed, and they need further debate and deliberation.

2. Fetal and maternal interactions There is increasing evidence that the period of intra-uterine growth is crucial for subsequent health—not just short-term health at the time of delivery or in infancy, but long term and into adulthood. If these early results of research are confirmed then the long-term consequences for the population as a whole will be considerable. There are many factors involved in this interaction including smoking, radiation, drugs, viruses, and the nutritional status of the mother.

3. Behaviour change and mental health Much of ill health is determined by our behaviour, generally freely chosen. Some of these choices are due to lack of information, but for most people this is not the case. Few can be unaware of the dangers of cigarette smoking, drug abuse, or drinking and driving. Yet in spite of this information the choices we make about healthy living may be the wrong ones. For this reason there is an urgent need to consider how we can better understand these issues.

Mental health issues are also of considerable importance; their impact and cost on individuals, families, and communities is significant. Included within this are matters of addiction such as drug misuse, alcohol abuse, and cigarette smoking. Greater effort and resources are required to be able to understand and deal with the problems in an effective way. It is encouraging to see that mental health is now at the top of the agenda for many organizations and agencies with an interest in health.

In terms of basic research, advances in the neurosciences and cognitive development are fascinating and likely, in the long term, to change our thinking and understanding of the workings of the mind.

4. Clinical practice

1. Developments in medicine and the diffusion of innovation It is assumed that new discoveries in diagnosis and treatment will continue to occur, often in an unpredictable way, and that the new technology will increasingly define the resources required. Further developments will come from a wide range of places, and the intelligence function must be alert to new ideas. On their own, however, these are not enough; ideas need to be put into practice. This 'diffusion of innovation' is critical and should be actively researched.

The consultation between the doctor and the patient as the building block of health care will assume even greater importance as the place where decision making about resources and clinical skills come together. The key issue for the future will be how quickly such advances can be introduced into clinical practice after an assessment of effectiveness has been made.

2. Evidence-based medicine This is here to stay, and it will be increasingly difficult in the future to introduce a treatment or procedure into routine clinical practice which has not been fully evaluated. This does not, and should not, inhibit research and development; it is not about 'cookbook' medicine. More and more there will be questioning of procedures and treatments to ensure their effectiveness. The outcome of care, and the quality of the care provided will be the driving force for change. Outcomes are difficult to measure in many clinical conditions but this will remain a major professional challenge. In the future clinical practice will be built on a combination of three factors: personal clinical experiences, linked to external sources of advice from databases, and, of increasing importance, input from patients. The importance of clinical skills in this process must be emphasized.

3. The role of information technology Information technology is one of the most rapidly developing aspects of health care. As the process become more user-friendly, so the possibilities become ever more exciting. So, ability to access databases for clinical work, increasing sophistication of diagnostic procedures, rapidity of sharing information, decision support facilities, and the use of the information 'superhighway' (the internet) all indicate the enormous potential for the use of computers and information management in the improvement of the health of the nation. Already patients are better informed and are able, from the wide range of resources available, to have access to information—often in advance of those in the clinical specialties.

One further important issue should be raised, and that is the confidentiality of information. As the technology advances, so this necessity must not be forgotten.

4. Ethical issues in health and health care Throughout this book the importance of ethical issues has been emphasized. The values which society gives to health determine the way in which individuals and the community will respond to information and initiatives. These values set the importance of health in context and give direction to ethical decisions which have to be made. Public debate and discussion, and a greater understanding of the scientific basis of health, are necessary if difficult ethical decisions are to be made.

5. Emergency services As the health of the population improves and chronic diseases are controlled more effectively, so the importance of emergency services will be increasingly recognized. These are at the front line of health services, and often are concerned with matters of life and death. Those involved, from the primary health care team through to the trauma centre, need effective training and support. The organization of such services requires careful consideration to meet the needs of the population and to provide a high-quality service, staffed with those with special experience and skills. Access to information and advice will be central to this and will require the skills to use information technology. The public also have a responsibility to ensure that they too are able to deal with emergencies, and have resuscitation and first aid skills.

5. Public health issues

1. The environment While the effects of the environment on health are increasingly recognized, the strength of the links between them needs to be developed further. There must be much more research in this area if we are to take full benefit from a cleaner environment. Environmental incidents of international significance are now with us and action plans to be able to deal with these are essential. The UK Environment and Health Action Plan (UKEHAP) puts the subject firmly on the agenda, and environment will feature within the 'Our Healthier Nation' strategy and will strengthen this even further.

2. Infectious disease Over the last few years we have seen how the changing pattern of infection has challenged the scientific community. New infections, and old ones in new disguises, have appeared with significant threats to human health. Such new organisms as prions and HIV infection are major problems to understand and control. The capacity to keep up with such developments must not be lost.

A specific subset of this is the internationally recognized problem of antibiotic-resistant micro-organisms. These are increasingly common and can have most serious consequences. Action will need to be taken to limit the range of organisms involved. This will have implications for human clinical practice, agriculture, fishing, and animal health.

3. Screening Already it is possible to screen for infection, childhood illnesses, and several cancers, and to take early action to deal with the problem. Quality control and an evaluation of effectiveness are essential if the programme is to improve health outcomes. Over the next few years a number of new screening programmes are likely to become available, and the developments in genetics will increase this. The practical problems of introducing such programmes are well-known, as are the ethical issues. However, the necessity for public debate is urgent, as is the need for a greater public understanding of the science behind screening.

4. Immunization The power and success of immunization are well-known. Vaccination procedures are perhaps the most cost effective of all interventions to improve and protect health. There is still more to be done, and there are a number of diseases which could be controlled or eradicated. The elimination of smallpox in the world showed what could be achieved, and we now need the worldwide disappearance of polio, measles, and others. New vaccine developments will make them even safer and will extend their range. Chickenpox, meningococcal meningitis, HIV infection, and many others may be within reach in the not too distant future.

The link between immunization and non-communicable disease should not be forgotten. For example, immunization against hepatitis B is likely to lead to a reduction in hepatocellular cancer, and it could eventually be possible to immunize against the virus which may cause cancer of the cervix.

5. *Violence* This is emerging as a major public health issue. Whether it relates to domestic violence, class or ethnic conflicts, or hostilities between nations, the impact is huge. In some circumstances it is the main constraint to improving public health.

6. *The role of the public* If the health of the nation is to be improved then public involvement is crucial. This has been discussed in detail in Chapter 4. However, it is worth reiterating the need to use the skills and resources of patients and the public in improving health and health care. The use of participation groups, citizens juries, community representatives, all have a role. The rapid development of information technology will see that they are very well provided for.

6. Some conclusions

The twenty or so issues raised here represent a personal view of some important topics for the future. It is essential that these are debated and discussed, and, more especially, changed, modified, and reviewed as new developments occur. The potential is limitless, and health can be improved.

14

Making it happen

'The prior knowledge of the learner is of crucial importance in the learning of any new concepts.'* Edgar Stone, *Psychology of education

1. Introduction

If we accept that education is a process, the chief aim of which is to bring about a change in behaviour, then 'making it happen', changing health, is about learning to think and act differently. As the quotation above makes clear, one of the most important things about learning is what the learner already knows. We must start therefore where individuals, communities, countries are in their development. We cannot, and should not, make assumptions about beliefs and attitudes. We need to understand where people are, and to facilitate change, not impose it. The educational quotation used, and an understanding of the role of teaching and learning are therefore apposite.

Further, if the concept behind this book is accepted—that is that much could be done with existing knowledge to improve health, and that the potential for doing so is enormous—then the real question which must be addressed is how can we make it happen? As usual there are a series of different audiences to which this question can be addressed —individuals, families, communities, workplaces and organizations, professionals, national government and international agencies. As has been said many times in this book, the key to releasing the potential is through people. The evidence is there that health can be improved, let's make it happen.

But how should I get started? What should I do on Monday morning? What action can I take now which will improve health? What lessons can be learnt and taken forward? Should I wait until more evidence is available? How much disruption will be caused? Will it cost much? These were all questions which were raised at the beginning of this book. Much of course depends on the particular problem to be faced. It should be clear from earlier discussions that many of the problems are complex, that there are no easy or simple answers, and that the evidence base may be weak or uncertain in some instances. Does this mean that I do nothing until the science base has been improved? Of course not. Enough is now known about health to realize a great deal of the potential. Most of the issues are about the management of change, and a huge amount has already been written on this subject. The following summarizes a very personal view of the literature:

1. Do you know what the problem is? Have you looked into the issue and are you sure of the facts? Take cigarette smoking as an example. Are you sure of all the evidence of the risks incurred in smoking?
2. On the basis of the information, do I (or does my organization) need to change? What would be the value of doing so? What are the difficulties in changing and what challenges would need to be faced?
3. What would be the costs to myself or my organization, not only in financial terms but at a personal level?
4. If I did change would my friends and workmates support me (or ridicule me)? Does the social context in which I live and work make it easy or difficult for me?
5. What would I actually need to do? Could I set myself a personal set of objectives to change? If I was the head of an organization could I specify these objectives and implement them? What would stop me?
6. If I did want to change how would I know that things had got better? Could I work out some measurable targets linked to the objectives?
7. Do I have sufficient people on board to help with any

change? People are the key to change. They need to be partners and to participate in the process. A significant amount of time may need to be invested with key people in convincing them of the need to change.

What is required is an action plan which ensure that health issues are not forgotten. Some of this was discussed in the chapter on the 'Art of public health'. The following outline **ACTION PLAN** may help to structure any initiative:

A. Agenda setting
Getting a health topic on the agenda can be difficult but is the key. Until the group, organization, committee, has agreed to this, then little can be done. The stages of getting there have already been described in Chapter 8.
C. Communicate effectively
Having got the subject on the agenda, it is crucial that the opportunity is not lost. A clear presentation of the issue and possible solutions is required.
T. Training and education
What are the skills required to deal with the issues? Are they available, or does more need to be done? Are the right people with the right skills in the right place?
I. Infrastructure
In any action plan there is a need for organizational issues to be tackled and effective networks established.
O. Operational issues
What are the tactics to be used? Are the resources available? Is the skills mix right?
N. Need for research
Are the right questions being asked? Can the research findings be implemented? Research and the development of the evidence is at the heart of the process.
P. Perception of risk
This is a major obstacle to the changing of health and lifestyle. How can health promotion programmes be more effective?
L. Leadership
This is necessary to manage the process of change. It requires an understanding of innovation and the changes

in practice which will occur as a result of new developments. It needs to have a clear ethical framework and value base.

A. Audit and evaluation

This involves monitoring, information systems, and the critical use of databases.

N. National responsibility

Health is everyone's responsibility. All must be concerned to play their part in improving health.

2. Change at different levels

The personal level

In some ways, changing yourself is the most difficult task. Early on in this book the question was raised, what's in it for me? If I do change my eating or my smoking will it be worthwhile? Will the pain be worth the gain? Will the investment be worth it? It is hoped that the book has shown how, with relatively small changes in lifestyle, much can be achieved. Here are some pointers based on what we already know and have discussed throughout the book. They are given for advice only and are not meant to be nannying. It is for you to make the choices:

1. Enjoy life. Being healthy is a good thing to be, not bad. Health is a positive concept, and quality of life and how you feel about yourself is at the heart of this. Keeping yourself healthy is about doing good things, as well as the occasional 'don't'.
2. Take regular, moderate exercise, in keeping with your age and medical condition. The benefits of exercise are considerable, affecting the heart, lungs, muscle function, and bone strength. It also makes you feel good.
3. Enjoy your food. Take a balanced, varied diet. Keep your weight under control.
4. Feeling good about yourself is not easy in a changing world with the increasing pace of life and the associated stress. Yet this is very much part of feeling healthy. Make

sure you have some quiet time for yourself on a regular basis, and ensure that you have someone to talk to when necessary. Men, in particular, seem to have more difficulty in talking things over with others. See your doctor if you have concerns about your health.

5. Sexual health is also important in a full and healthy life. The advice on safe sex is well-known and is highly relevant for those who change partners.
6. You have a contribution to make to the health of your family, your circle of friends, and the wider community. you should put into practice the lessons learned, and consider your role in making the community in which you live more healthy, with a clean and safe environment. Being a good parent would be part of this.
7. Look after yourself if you have an illness—it's part of your responsibilities. Make sure you see your doctor if you are concerned.
8. Enjoy the sunshine, but take precautions by wearing appropriate clothes and sun screens.
9. Injuries can often be prevented. Look out for things around the home, at work and at leisure which may result in injury. Take particular care with children and the elderly. Do a regular "accident" check at home and at work.
10. The serious health consequences of smoking cigarettes, taking drugs, and drinking and driving are well-known. The evidence is clear and the health benefits of *not* smoking, taking drugs, or drinking and driving are real. The choice is yours.

There is nothing very revolutionary in the ten points listed. If everyone was to change even a little, then the health of the population would increase and people would feel better. For each individual, of course, there is no guarantee that following the advice just given will banish illness and disability. But the chances of improving quality of life will increase.

The difficulty in changing behaviour or lifestyle depends on the importance, or the value, of the change. This 'value-based learning' suggests that change only occurs if the value of the change is greater than the present situation. For example, someone who smokes cigarettes may opt to continue smoking (in spite of being aware of all the evidence for its harmful effects) because the benefits of smoking are perceived to be greater than stopping. The hypothesis then suggests that a change in behaviour will only occur if this is reversed. Giving information, or even advice may not be enough. The person needs to want to change. This is why emphasis has been placed on the individual asking the question of themselves, what will be the value of this change to me?

There is considerable debate on whether changing behaviour is more dependent on the individual or the environment. Both are clearly important, but there is little doubt that to change personal behaviour in a hostile environment can be very difficult.

Much has been mentioned in the press about the problems of 'nannying', by which, it is assumed, is generally meant to imply telling people what to do against their better judgement. The Oxford English Dictionary gives one definition of the word 'nanny' as 'an unduly protective person or institution'. In relation to health, the giving of information and advice does not seem to come into this category. Neither does explaining what influences health and the consequences to the individual of lifestyle factors. It is the difference between saying 'don't smoke' (nannying) and outlining the serious health consequences of smoking (information giving), from which the individual can make a choice. That said, however, it is necessary that information is given and clearly presented, and in a form which is understandable, and that those who wish advice (as opposed to simply information) are given it. Those who disagree with the advice have a right to say so, but they should not call giving information 'nannying'.

The same principles apply to populations and to public health measures. For example, immunization of the population as a whole is a highly effective method of reducing the burden of childhood infectious diseases. Consent however is required, and must be given. The consequences of not being immunized need to be clearly and unambiguously laid out, as well as the possible side-effects. As has been emphasized throughout this book, information needs to be based on evidence, and counter-arguments require the same degree of rigour.

The family

The family remains a very powerful focus for learning about health. Social and personal behaviour is acquired within the family (and in other settings of course); eating habits and other lifestyle issues are all parts of family life. Young children, adolescents, adults, and, with the extended family, elderly people, can all contribute to being a healthy family. Parenting skills, for those who have less support around them, might be one way of ensuring that appropriate experience and expertise in raising families are developed. As most health care is self-care, the family level is where most of this is done. Just as professional staff have a responsibility for ensuring that they are up to date, so it should be for those who make decisions about the health of relatives and friends.

The school

The concept of the healthy school is now well recognized, and includes taking particular care with the environment and with the food provided. It is concerned with supporting children, and with creating a culture where the problems of smoking, drugs, alcohol, and sexual health can be readily discussed, and advice given.

The community

Improving the health of the population as a whole is the responsibility of many different groups—the public, professionals, politicians, faith groups, special interest groups, voluntary organizations, international agencies, and so on. The potential is there to make a major impact on health and improve the quality of life of the community. This is not just about health services—an important but limited way of changing the health of large numbers of people—but it is about education, the role of women, the environment, transport, food, air and water quality, provided in a safe place, free from violence. There are some very exciting community development projects around the country which show just how much energy and enthusiasm is available. The potential is enormous if we are only able to free up the creativity of the population. Health action zones and healthy living centres are part of this.

The workplace

The workplace is an important setting for improving health, a key element of which is ensuring the safety of the workforce. A business with a low illness and absence rate will be more efficient and more productive. There is a real challenge for organizations to improve health by first recognizing its importance (getting it on the agenda). The provision of good healthy eating choices, no smoking areas, advice on drugs and alcohol, and an occupational health service can go a very long way towards better health. Exercise and recreational facilities and the availability of a creche, if they can be provided, can help even further with creating a healthy workforce. Good health is good business.

The professionals Throughout this book the necessity for professional staff to think about health, as well as illness, has been emphasized. This is an important responsibility and much could be done during routine consultations to give advice, to encourage healthier lifestyles, and to help people make choices. Professionals are major role models.

In many instances it will be the health professionals—doctors, nurses, dentists, and so on—who will be the leaders of the process of change and the agents who will facilitate it. This essential role will be discussed in more detail later in this chapter.

At the national level The importance of developing cross-departmental national health plans is a central part of the long-term objective of improving health. The determinants of health—genetics, socio-economic factors (including education, lifestyle, the environment), and the health service—make it clear that improving health is not about one sector of the country or one organization, but concerns a very wide range of individuals, groups, and organizations. Partnership and teamwork are crucial. Community development projects in which the whole community works together to achieve a common objective are good examples of this. The 'Health For All' strategy of the WHO set the tone, and this has been adapted by many countries as a national health policy. In England, the 'Our Healthier Nation' strategy is one such interdepartmental national health plan, which has a small number of key areas and targets. This initiative is supplemented by the National Environment and Health Action Plan.

At the international level In addition to the WHO, a wide range of other agencies have an interest in improving health. Collaboration between them is essential if the best use is to be made of the resources available. Disease is no respecter of country or continent. The quality of the land, the air, and the waters of the world, are all vital if health is to be maintained. Communicable disease can spread rapidly, and unexpectedly, and there is a need for surveillance mechanisms to give early warning signs of problems. Radiation incidents can affect large numbers of the population and, in such instances, the need for co-ordinated action becomes paramount. The WHO plays a leading part in all this.

3. Leadership

Much of the evidence suggests that if change is to be effective, leadership is essential. Leaders, role models, and peer group leaders all have a significant impact on shaping behaviour, both of individuals and groups. Their importance in being able to tell stories and to develop a clear vision has been described in Chapter 10.

It is often said of a good teacher that, for the pupils, the subject is 'caught, not taught'. The good teacher facilitates, and his or her infectious enthusiasm seems to be able to change others. This 'contagious theory of behaviour change' is not new. History shows how individuals have influenced the lives of others, and, even now, role models are very powerful in setting trends in behaviour, style, clothes, and attitudes. People of all ages (not just the young) need someone to relate to and who can set an example. The role of the doctor (as a powerful role model) in assisting patients to stop smoking is well-known, as is the role of the footballer, pop star, or personality. Such individuals tell good stories (in words or deeds) and set examples. Courage, fear, enthusiasm, and a wish to change are all infectious.

In changing health, we need committed people who want to make things better—at local level, at group level, within the community, at national level. Many of these will be health professionals. Within organizations and families, leadership is essential. But change also requires a strong commitment to education and to providing opportunities for the natural enthusiasm and creativity of individuals and the community to be expressed.

4. The future

Change can happen. The potential is there; it just needs to be realized. It is the responsibility of us all to ensure it does happen. Changing health for the better is not a short-term issue; the results may not be seen for many years. Yet the need to begin the process is evident. It's a little like planting a tree. It will take many years to fulfil its promise, but the very act of planting is a significant one. Planting the seeds of good health in the younger generation will lead to better health in the long term. In years to come, future generations will not count our progress by the number of reports and papers we have written, but by what we achieved. In the words of St Matthew 'By their fruits ye shall know them'. It is by our fruits that others will judge our efforts.

Further reading

Stones, E. (1983). *Psychology of education*. Methuen, London.

15

Envoi

'Life is short, and the art long; the occasion fleeting, experience fallacious, and judgement difficult. The physician must not only be prepared to do what is right himself, but also to make the patient, the attendants, and externals co-operate.'
Hippocrates

The process of bringing together this book, coupled with a look towards the future, encourages a more philosophical and personal view to be put forward at this stage. The book has identified a series of broad general themes, which it might be worth reviewing, and these include:

1. Health, and the potential to improve it, is associated with many other issues—education, social factors, employment, housing, peace and security, and the environment being some. Health and sustainable development, and health and the ecological dimension are closely linked.

2. Health is very much a political issue (with a big 'P' and a small 'p'), and will not change unless those who have political power at all levels wish it to do so and the population want it to happen and see value in it. Almost all change is wrought through people, as individuals and as groups. The particular role of women in the process of improving health has been emphasized many times in this book.

3. The changes which are required are based on the available knowledge of how health can be improved. Thus research and the gaining of new and improved evidence is essential. The knowledge base is, of course, increasing all the time, but at times it is not sufficicent to make effective

decisions. It is for this reason that judgement will still be necessary in order to make decisions in the face of uncertainty. This implies that the values and ethical base of those who make such judgements is clear and explicit. Values are therefore the single most important factor in improving health.

4. Participation and involvement of patients and the public is fundamental. The power of communities to change health and to improve their environment is impressive when it is seen in action. We need to do all we can to encourage such ownership. Part of this is the role of education in improving the ability of individuals to make choices and to act in a positive way in relation to health. Educational attainment is one of the key determinants of health.

5. It is sometimes assumed that longevity is the appropriate outcome for improved health. This may not always be the case, and improved quality of life may be just as important, or more so. It is perhaps the real goal. In his book, *What kind of life*, Daniel Callaghan explores this issue and asks about the purpose of health. Is it a means or an end? This issue has been discussed earlier in this book. It is however a fundamental question. Why do we want to be healthy, and what levels of ill health or disability can or should be tolerated in any society? Hans Kung, in *Global responsibility*, asks the same kind of question, seeking an answer which is a balance between different views. It is a question which needs to be asked, though it will be difficult to answer. Perhaps there is not a single 'answer' to be found, but instead it is simply a process of continual striving to make things better for more of the people more of the time.

6. In clinical terms, the medical profession, and other professional groups, need to look ahead and respond to change. They must provide clear leadership and emphasize the importance of values, quality, clinical skills, management, an holistic approach and the need for co-operation

and teamwork. They should continually recognize the power of patient participation, and be at the leading edge of encouraging full involvement.

7. Inequities and inequalities exist; it is not difficult to demonstrate them. The question is what to do about them. This is not an easy issue and will require leadership and commitment. The words of Martin Luther King ring true:

> Human progress is neither automatic or inevitable . . . Every step towards the goal of social justice requires sacrifice, suffering and struggle, and the passionate concerns of dedicated individuals . . . This is no time for apathy or complacency. This is a time for vigorous and positive action.

But it is people who are the salvation. It is by people and through people that the gains are to be won. In spite of all of the pressures in this late twentieth century, people still want to help others, and see within that purpose something worthwhile and valuable:

> A man is never so well employed as when he is labouring for the advantage of the public; without the expectation, the hope, or even the wish to derive any advantage of any kind from the results of his exertions. Sir Joseph Banks

> How selfish soever man may be supposed, there are evidently some principles in his nature, which interest him in the fortunes of others, though he derives nothing from it but the pleasure of seeing it. Adam Smith

These two quotations, coupled with the one from Martin Luther King, stress the goodness of the human spirit, and the importance of public service.

In coming to the end of this book, three different analogies suggest themselves, which might illustrate the ways forward. The first is a golf analogy, and seeks to compare my golf with that of Jack Nicklaus. I am small and dark, and he is tall and blond. But these are not the only differences. He plays golf regularly, and I don't. He has a full set of clubs, and I don't. He is in fact very good at golf, and I'm very much the amateur. But the main difference between us is that when he plays golf he plays to win, and when I play golf I am just so glad to get on to the fairway that I don't care if I win or lose. And here is the analogy. Health will be improved by those who practise regularly, who have a full set of clubs, who can get out of bunkers when they need to, who are good at it, but most of all, who want to win.

The second is a nautical analogy. Consider a large tanker sailing in the ocean, needing to change direction. It can be difficult to do this, but it can be done, and made much easier if a series of small but powerful tug boats assist. We have such tug boats to change the direction of health. They are the individuals and organizations with the skills knowledge, and experience to move the tanker of health.

The third analogy comes from thermodynamics and is concerned with the nature of entropy. Here are some definitions:

- energy is the capacity to do work
- when work is done, energy is transformed from one form into another
- energy is therefore stored work
- power is the rate at which work is done
- disorder always tends to increase—entropy increases—when no work is done
- energy is required to restore order

The significance of these statements is, I hope, obvious. There is a need for energy, power, and work if disorder is to be controlled. The natural tendency in the physical world (and I suspect in the biological world) is to disorder—entropy. But it can be prevented and reversed.

These three analogies make three separate points. First, we can win, but it will require skill, practice, and commitment. It is not a part-time task. Second, this will be helped if we all pull together, and in the same direction. Finally, such change will only come about if energy and enthusiasm are there in abundance.

The world is a remarkable place—ice, deserts, forests, seas, villages, towns, and cities. Human beings have an enormous potential to adapt to all of these conditions, giving a diversity and richness to life. With the goodwill of people, wanting to improve the common weal, then health can and will be improved.

Further reading

Callaghan, D. (1995). *What kind of life: the limits of medical progress.*
Kung, H. (1990). *Global responsibility: in search of a new world ethic.* SCM Press, Edinburgh.

Subject Index

abortion 147
accidents
  childhood 24–5
  emergency services 177, 214, 249
  Health of the Nation strategy 46
  perceptions of health 60–1
  variations in health 35
adolescents 51, 132, 192–3
advertising
  'add an egg' storyline 56
  international health 146
age factors 244
  see also adolescents; children; elderly people
AIDS and HIV 14, 36, 47, 59, 90, 142
alienation 40–3, 92
Alma-Ata declaration 30
anaesthesia 11
antibiotics 11, 65, 250
antisepsis 11
art/s 97–104
  in hospitals 101–2
  in medical education 103, 230
  of medicine 17–18, 66, 97
  of public health 118–27
  see also literature
asthma 159–60
attitude change 63
audiovisual presentations 180
audit, clinical 157, 164–8, 204, 255
autonomy 89, 97

behavioural issues 246–7
  'contagious theory' 261
  future issues 117
  knowledge/perceptions 60–1, 65
  lifestyle 5, 14, 33, 54
  research into 132, 134
  role models 63, 259–61
  see also change and innovation
beneficence 89, 176
biochemical factors 134–5
Black Report 45
body language 67, 179, 180
breast cancer 51 (*Fig.*), 52, 77
breast milk substitute 147
British Medical Association
  Living with risk 62, 86
building standards 10

cancer 73–6
  breast 51 (*Fig.*), 52, 77
  Expert Advisory Group 241
  Health of the Nation strategy 46
  lung 24, 51 (*Fig.*), 53, 94, 142
  mortality 50–1 (*Figs*), 53, 142
  a problem still 66
  registration 73–6
  specialization 210, 211, 213–14
  variations in health 36
caring 150, 176, 180
Certificate of Completion of Specialist Training (CCST) 211, 228
change and innovation 252–62
  ACTION PLAN 21, 249, 254–5, 260
  attitudes 63
  community level 18, 258–9
  diffusion of 247
  doctors' interest in 205
  educational basis 3, 21, 64, 254
  energy/enthusiasm for 266
  ethical basis 3, 21
  facilitate rather than impose 252
  family level 258
  international level 260
  management of 26–9, 121 252–62
  models for 64
  national level 260
  personal level 63, 255–8
  poverty 44
  professional level 259
  public health 118, 120–3
  reasons for 123
  research basis 3, 17, 21, 64, 254
  responsibility for 18–19, 121
  school level 258
  society level 63–4
  timing of 64, 152
  tools for changing perceptions 63–5
  workplace level 259
  see also behavioural issues; leadership

children
  accidents 24–5
  adolescents 51, 132, 192–3
  Health of the Young Nation 53
  infant mortality 10, 110, 140–1, 166
  Our Healthier Nation strategy 53
  perceptions of health 62
  schools 53, 258
  UNICEF 138
clinical audit 157, 164–8, 204, 255
Clinical Outcomes Group 167
clinical standards 157–9, 165–9, 204, 235
clinical trials 162–3
communication 178–82
  of bad news 179, 181
  doctors' ability 200, 205
  education and training 233
  and the humanities 103
  of information/intelligence 68, 71, 110
  management of change 254
  new Hippocratic 'promise' 219–20
  non–verbal 67, 179
  of risk 71–83, 94
  skill of 67–8, 181–2
  teamwork 239–40
  verbal 179
  written 180
community 28, 258–9
  arts 102
  development projects 28, 44, 50, 259–60
  health councils 19, 57
  involvement in change 18, 258–9
  leaders 29
  medical schools 230
  needs and expectations 7, 14
  population growth/size 12, 147
  rights 88–90
  'therapeutic' 241
  see also patients and public; society
computers 68, 177–8, 248
Confidential Enquiries 166
confidentiality 166, 240, 248
consensus 39, 163
consultations 184, 200, 247
continuing medical education (CME) 205, 228–9, 234
continuing professional development (CPD) 203, 212–13, 228–9
contraception 77–8, 147
coronary problems, *see* heart disease
costs and economics
  international variations in health 142–3
  opportunity costs 69
  prevention of illness 128–9
  prosperity and health 10–11
  recession 141
  treatment costs 70, 94
  see also income; resources; socio-economic factors
Council of Europe 148
creativity 26–7, 182
  see also art/s
Creutzfeldt-Jakob disease (CJD) 24
cultural issues 18, 90, 131
  see also ethnic minorities; socio-economic factors
curriculum, *see* medical education and training

data analysis/collection, *see* information and intelligence
decision making
  distributive justice 36–7
  ethical base 88, 92–3, 95
  patient choice 67–71
  see also resources
dementia 24, 191
Department of Health
  Chief Medical Officer 114, 124
  Variations in health 36, 45, 48
deprivation 40–1, 92
  see also socio-economic factors
diabetes 6
disabled people 194–5, 244
disease
  classification of 11
  communicable 33, 138–9, 142
    see also infectious disease/s
  components of 6
  'compression' of morbidity 7, 244–5
  diagnosis of 11, 65–6, 106, 200–1, 221
  hereditary 111
    see also genetic issues
  lowering morbidity rate 14
  models of 206
  and outcome of health care 16
  prevention of 127–31
  prognosis 106–7, 200
  treatment factors 16, 66, 70, 77–8, 94, 200
  understanding of 11, 246–7
  see also individual diseases
doctors
  career advice 216
  characteristics of 202–5, 209–12, 224–5

civil service 124
derivation of word 232
fallibility of 66
fictional 224
generalists v. specialists 214, 234
overseas 212
problem 168, 235
quality of 157
range of 225
specialist, *see* specialization/ specialties
teaching role 221
Tomorrow's doctors 84, 227
trust in 167, 232
see also professional issues
donor agencies 147, 148
drugs 144, 146

economics, *see* costs and economics
education
determinant of health 5, 10, 34, 132
international variations in health 143
management 236
professional, *see* medical education and training
public 176
elderly people 53, 142, 191–2, 244
emergency services 177, 214, 249
endocrinological factors 134–5
environmental issues 5, 12, 33, 139
UKEHAP 249, 260
epidemics 139
epidemiology 115, 131
behavioural 132
cancer studies 74, 75
cellular 135
molecular 117, 135
equality/equity 34–9, 91–2
distinctions between them 35
international health 146
resource allocation 68
see also Health for All; health inequalities; justice
ethical issues 19–20, 87–96
basis of change 3, 21
differences of opinion 96
evolutionary 90
future concerns 248–9
genetics 94, 111–12
Hippocratic Oath 9, 197, 216–23, 263
humanities 97
information/intelligence 111–12
international health 89, 145–8
'my mother' principle 97
poverty 43
public debate 89
research ethics committees 85
resource allocation 174
teaching medical ethics 96
see also risk; values
ethnic minorities 49, 61, 147–8
Europe 22, 140–2, 148
evaluation
information/intelligence 106
interventions 21, 36, 133
management of change 255
quality of care 155–7, 165, 206
specialist services 215
evidence-based medicine 3, 162–4, 248
art of public health 119–20
resource allocation 175
risk communication 75
value of specialization 210
exercise 51–2, 255

fairness, *see* equality/equity
family issues 27, 245, 258
fetal–maternal interactions 109, 246
food poisoning/safety 60, 136

General Medical Council (GMC)
establishment of 13
medical education/registration 226–7
specialist register 211, 228
and standards 158–9, 235
Tomorrow's doctors 84, 227
general practice, *see* primary care
genetic issues
determinants of health 5, 32–3, 246
ethical issues 94, 111–12
future concern 117
global issues 22, 93, 146, 264
see also international health
guidelines 163, 204–5

hazards 76–7
Health Alliance Awards 50
health and health care
access to 132
action zones 54
agenda setting 254
UN Agenda 21 strategy 5, 33, 139
compassion 150, 176, 180
comprehensive health service 175–7

health and health care (*cont.*)
definitions 4–5, 8, 31–2, 114–15, 150–1
determinants 5–6, 10, 21, 32–4, 132, 246
see also education; socio-economic factors
developing countries 139, 144–7
see also international health
disabled people 194–5, 244
doctors' concern with 204
ecological approach 8
economic aspects, *see* costs and economics
effectiveness 159–63, 204, 210
elderly people 53, 142, 191–2, 244
emergency services 177, 214, 249
entropy analogy 266
in Europe 22, 140–2, 148
expectations of 7, 14, 64–6
facilities 16, 174
see also hospitals; resources
future issues 116–17, 130, 243–51, 260–2
global, *see* international health
golf analogy 265–6
historical issues 8–15, 42, 139, 231–2
holistic approach, *see* holism
hospital-based 49, 101–2, 177, 211
and the humanities, *see* art/s
improvement of 1–2
see also change and innovation
intersectoral issues 8, 143
investment in 147
limits to 13
long–term 192
and the media 64, 72, 82–3, 178
'memories' 185–8
men 50–1, 62, 193
mental 36, 46, 142, 190–1, 246–7
monitoring 3, 65, 158–9
see also evaluation; information and intelligence
multidisciplinary approach, *see* teamwork
occupational 28, 50–4, 259
organizational issues 207, 213–14, 254
see also management
palliative 160
partnerships 31–2, 51, 148
patient involvement, *see* patients and public
'Pepsi concept' 5
perceptions of 60–5, 254
potential for 1–2, 252–3
predicting 22, 109–10
primary, *see* primary care
professionals, *see* professional issues
public education on 176
public involvement, *see* patients and public
public understanding of 85
purpose of 6–8, 32, 153
quality of, *see* quality of care; quality of life
rationing 14
see also resources
reproductive 146–7
responsibility for 18–19, 31, 121, 151, 255
see also 'health by all'
sexual 36, 47, 256
special services, *see* specialization/ specialties;
staff, *see* professional issues
standards 10, 157–8, 165–9, 204
statistics 140
see also information and intelligence
structure of 177
see also organizational issues
surveillance 3, 65, 158–9
see also evaluation; information and intelligence
'tales and legends' 182–5
technology, *see* health technology assessment; information technology
'ten commandments' 27
theories of 206
tugboat analogy 266
value of 92–3
variations, *see* health inequalities
workplace 28, 50–4, 259
see also children; communication; community; cultural issues; disease; ethical issues; medical education and training; medicine; models; national issues; outcome issues; policy issues; public health; research; risk; targets; women
health and safety 10, 28
see also occupational health
'health by all' 3, 19, 31, 47, 255
Health for All 2, 30–1, 34–9, 145, 260
health inequalities 7, 25, 265
hospital outcomes 162
international variations 138–49
research effort 133–5
Variations in health 36, 45, 48

see also equality/equity; Health for All; Health of the Nation strategy; socio-economic factors
Health of the Nation strategy 31, 46–54
Health of the Young Nation 50
'Our Healthier Nation' 19, 44, 46, 53, 131, 260
health professionals, *see* professional issues
health promotion 127–8
health status 16, 138, 160
health technology assessment 109, 164
healthy alliances 49
healthy groups 49
healthy living centres 54
healthy schools 258
healthy settings 48
heart disease
bypass surgery 69
factors involved 6
inequalities 36
mortality 51 (*Fig.*), 66, 141
Hippocrates/Hippocratic Oath 9, 197, 216–23, 263
new 'promise' 219–23
historical issues 8–15, 42, 139, 231–2
HIV and AIDS 14, 36, 47, 59, 90, 142
holism
definition of health 5, 8, 32
in diagnosis 200–1
health care and compassion 150, 176, 180
and humanities 103
new Hipporcratic 'promise' 222
specialist cancer services 213
hospitals 49, 101–2, 177, 211
housing 9, 12, 131
humanitarian agencies 148
humanities, *see* art/s
hygiene 136–7

immigration 131, 139
immunization 11, 33, 142, 250, 257–8
immunological factors 134–5
income 41–3, 131
see also poverty
individuals
changing health 63, 255–8
expectations and needs 7, 14
lifestyle factors 5, 14, 33, 54
rights of 88–9
role in health/care 26–7
values 90–1
infant mortality 10, 110, 140–1, 166
infectious disease/s 10, 33, 65, 138–9, 142, 249–50
see also AIDS and HIV; tuberculosis
information and intelligence 105–12
advice 257
collection of 9–10, 107, 200
communicating 67–8, 71, 110
consistency of 63
credibility of 72
evaluated 106
model of health/care 22
networks 108
patient involvement 68, 112
Public Health Common Data Set 47
routine 107, 160
sources of 108
systematizing 107
transfer 177
uncertainty 66, 74, 80, 82, 87–8
versus 'nannying' 257
see also knowledge; research
information technology 68, 177–8, 248
innovation, *see* change and innovation
international health 138–49
developing countries 139, 144–7
donor agencies 147, 148
ethical issues 89, 145–8
Europe 140–2, 148
factors in variations 140, 142–4
future issues 260
global issues 22, 93, 146, 264
medical fellowship 219
partnerships 31–2, 49, 148

Joint Committee for Training in General Practice 226
jurisprudence 37
justice 36–9, 45, 89
see also equality/equity

knowledge
advancing medical 17–18
and behaviour 59–60, 64
medical curriculum 205–6
perceptions of health 60–5
see also evidence-based medicine; information and intelligence; research

leadership 29, 185, 206–7
community leaders 29
managing change 173, 254–5, 260–1
teams 172, 238

learning, *see* medical education and training
legislation 90
life expectancy/lifespan 140–1, 153–4, 264
  see also mortality
lifelong learning 226, 228
lifestyle 5, 14, 33, 51
literature 97
  detectives 106
  fictional doctors 224
  and medicine 98–101, 230
  review of 184
lung cancer 24, 51, 53 (*Fig.*), 94, 142

management 169–73
  of change 26–9, 121 252–62
  education for 236
  and humanities 103–4
  of incidents 110–11
  models of 170–1
  professions in 171–3, 206
  of risk/uncertainty 87–8
  science 115
  and standards of care 158
  style 172
  'supermarket' model 170
marginalization 40–1
  see also socio–economic factors
maternal–fetal interactions 109, 246
maternal mortality 141, 142, 166
media 64, 72, 82–3, 178
medical education and training 224–37
  basis of change 3, 21, 63–4, 254
  and clinical audit 165–6
  communication skills 233
  continuing (CME) 205, 228–9, 234–5
  curriculum 91, 205–6, 225, 230–1
  in ethics 96
  future developments 236–7, 245
  in humanities 103, 230
  lifelong learning 226, 228
  in management 236
  and manpower 228
  multidisciplinary 98, 230, 240
  new Hippocratic 'promise' 220–1
  part–time 212
  patient involvement 83–5
  peer review 157, 169, 236
  postgraduate 227–8
  primary care 212, 226
  problem–based 230
  re–accreditation 234
  research in 232
  self–directed learning 228, 231
  specialists 211–16, 226–8
  team 240
  undergraduate 226–7
  values 91, 224
medical ethics, *see* ethical issues
medical giants 182
medical research, *see* research
medicine 198–207
  academic 116, 118, 211–12
  'art' of 17–18, 66, 97
  evolving 205
  fragmentation of 207
  future developments 207–16, 247
  international fellowship 219
  and literature 98–101, 230
  and public health 118
  public understanding of 85–7
  purpose of 198–9
  role of 197–207
  women in 227
  see also evidence–based medicine; health and health care; professional issues; specialization/specialties
men's health 61, 193
mental health 36, 46, 142, 190–1, 246–7
meta–analysis 163
metabolic factors 135
migration 12, 139, 141
models
  biological 170–1
  cancer services 213–14
  for change 63–4
  of health and illness 20–6, 38–9, 115, 206, 213
  of management 170–1
  'operatic' 170
  problem-based 63, 230
  role 62, 224–5, 259–61
  specialist training 211, 213–14
  'supermarket' 170
molecular biology 115, 117, 134–5, 246
moral issues, *see* ethical issues
morbidity, *see* disease
mortality
  'Bills of' 10, 34
  cancer 51–3, 52–3 (*Figs*), 142
  heart disease 51 (*Fig.*), 65, 141
  infant 10, 110, 140–1, 166
  lowering of 14
  male 193
  maternal 141, 142, 166
  see also life expectancy/lifespan

multimedia technology 178
music 97, 101–2

national issues 22, 28–9, 46–54, 260
  interdepartmental strategies 260
  NHS 12, 48, 49
  specialist services 177
  survey material 133
  see also Health of the Nation strategy
need 14
neurobiology 134
non–malevolence 89, 221
nutrition 59–60, 136

occupational health 28, 53–4, 259
occupational status 131
oral contraceptives 76–7
organizational issues 207, 213–14, 254
  see also management
'Our Healthier Nation' policy 19, 44, 46, 53, 131, 260
outcome issues 3, 15–17
  Clinical Outcomes Group 167
  and effectiveness 159–62, 204–5
  model for health/care 21
  specialist care 210

palliative care 160
parenting skills 258
patients and public 18, 55–86, 95, 206, 251, 264
  advocacy 68
  and the arts 102
  books written by 99
  choice in health care 68–70
  clinical audit process 167
  confidence in professionals 167, 232
  consent 84
  debate on ethical issues 89
  decision-making 88, 92–3, 95
  education on health 176
  empowerment 56
  focus of medicine 204
  ownership 56
  perceptions of health 60–4
  representation of 57–8
  role in information/intelligence 68, 112
  role in medical research 83–5
  role in professional education 83–5
  role in public health 251
  role in specialist services 215
  role in teamwork 241
  uncertainty 65–6, 74, 82, 87–8
  understanding of science etc 85
  see also adolescents; children; communication; disabled people; elderly people; ethnic minorities; family issues; individuals; men; society; women
peer groups 62, 260
peer review 157, 169, 236
personal issues, *see* individuals
pharmaceuticals 146
philosophy 97, 263
policy issues 38, 46
  Health for All 2, 30–1, 34–9, 145, 260
  UN Agenda 21
  strategy 5, 33, 139
  see also Health of the Nation strategy
political issues 19, 47, 63, 90, 115, 263
population
  growth/size 12, 147
  see also community; epidemiology
poverty 33, 39–44, 92, 142–3
  see also socio-economic factors
prenatal factors 109, 132, 246
prevention of illness 127–31
primary care 189–90
  bedrock of British health care 12–13
  comprehensive health service 176
  education and training 212, 226
  gatekeeping function 189, 234
  Health of the Nation strategy 48
  international health 144
  role in 'Health for All' 31
  and specialist cancer services 213
  teams 189–90
priority setting 14, 70
professional issues 197–242
  arrogance 220
  'bedside manner' 84
  competence 157, 231–6
  continuing development (CPD) 203, 212–13, 228–9
  'curiosity motive' 17, 27, 105
  definition of profession 199
  education, *see* medical education and training
  future action 207, 243–51, 261–2
  'grand rounds' 184
  Hippocratic Oath 9, 197, 216–23, 263
  listening 178, 179
  medicine as profession 198–207
  mentoring 168–9, 236

multiprofessional approaches, *see* teamwork
non-medical professions 215
organization/regulation 207, 213–14
performance review 157, 164, 167–9, 231–6
personal experiences 184
professionals in health/care 18–19, 27, 199–202, 259
skill mix 16, 237
skills as resources 16, 68–70, 174
teams, *see* teamwork
touching 180
values 91, 203–5
see also doctors; management; medicine; specialization/specialties
public health
and academia 118
art of 118–27
and clinical medicine 118
Common Data Set 47
comprehensive health service 176
current issues 116
data collection 10
definition of 114–15
equality/equity 38
ethical issues 87–96
future issues 116–17, 130, 249–51, 261–2
general principles 124–6
government role 122–4
Health of the Nation strategy 46
historical issues 9, 13
hitchhiker's guide to 126–7
improvements/initiatives in 120, 122
see also change and innovation
methodologies 116, 131–3
people skills 121
public role in 251
science of 114–18
teams 237–8
see also health and health care
public service 265

quality of care 154–9, 165, 206
quality of life 6–8, 130, 151–4, 244–5
definition of 6, 32
goal of improved health 264
improvement of 2
measuring 153
new Hippocratic 'promise' 219

racial factors 49, 62, 147–8
randomized clinical trials 162–3
rationing 14
Red Cross 148
rehabilitation 195
religious factors 147–8
reproductive health 146–7
research 127–36
basis of change 3, 17, 21, 63, 254
and development 63, 177, 205, 222
ethics committees 84
medical education 232
methodologies 116, 131–6
see also epidemiology
new Hippocratic 'promise' 222
poverty 43
role of public in 83–5
socio-economic approach to prevention 127–31
specialization in 205, 211–12, 215
teamwork 135–6, 240
see also information and intelligence; knowledge
resources
allocation 68–70, 90, 147, 173–7, 201
finite nature of 14
interpretation of 16, 69–70, 174
risk 71–82
absolute 76
assessment 74–7
benefit analysis 79–80
classification of 78–81
ethical issues 94
language of 72, 78–82
management of 87–8
perception 61, 254
relative 76
role models 62, 224–5, 259–61
Royal Colleges 158–9, 228
Royal Society
Risk analysis, perception and management 61, 86
rural areas 49

sanitation 10
schools 53, 258
science 114–18
certainty in 65–6, 74, 82, 87–8
new Hippocratic 'promise' 222
public understanding of 85
see also evidence-based medicine
screening 5, 117, 164, 250
self-care 3, 258
self-help groups 68

sexual health 36, 47, 256
smoking 14, 24, 59, 76, 142
society
caring 150, 176, 180
values of 90
see also community; patients and public
socio-economic factors 117, 243–5
determinants of health 5, 32–4, 128
historically 9, 12, 14
immunological consequences 134
poverty 33, 39–44, 92, 142–3
and prevention of illness 127–31
see also costs and economics; health inequalities
sociology 115
specialization/specialties 177, 189–96, 207–16
cancer 210, 211, 213–14
characteristics of 209–10
co-operation 207
disadvantages of 214
education and training 211–16, 226–8
evaluation of 215
non-medical professions 215
organization of 213–14
research 211–12, 215
role of public 215
specialist register 211, 228
Specialist Training Authority (STA) 211, 226, 228
value of 210
versus generalists 214, 234
standards 10, 157–8, 165–9, 204
stress 133–5, 196
stroke/s 36, 46
surgery outcomes 160

targets 17
Health for All strategy 145
Health of the Nation strategy 46–53, 55
model for health/care 21–2
WHO ethical 89
teaching, *see* medical education and training
teamwork 16–17, 204, 237–41
conflict 240
new Hippocratic 'promise' 221
primary care 189–90
public health 238
research 135–6, 240
specialists 209–10
team leaders 172, 238
team spirit 240
time factors
change 63, 152
income time lines 41–3
initiatives in public health 120
part-time education/training 212
as resource 69–70, 174
training, *see* medical education and training
tuberculosis 6, 142

UK Environment and Health Action Plan (UKEHAP) 249, 260
unemployment 196
United Nations
Agenda 21 strategy 5, 33, 139
Children's Fund (UNICEF) 138
utility 89, 97

vaccination 11, 33, 142, 250, 257–8
values 89–91
behaviour change 256–7, 264
educational 91, 224
health itself 92–3
hidden agenda 91, 205, 225
imposed 63
management 169
and perceptions of health 63
personal 90–1
political 90
professional 91, 203–5
quality of care 155
risk assessment 78–9
societal 90
of specialization 210
see also ethical issues
violence 132, 141, 143, 146, 251
voluntary sector 19

war 141, 143, 146
women 57, 193–4, 245
community change 18
educational status 143
historical trends 12
international health 142–3, 146–7
in medicine 227
perceptions of health 61
research into 132
'wise' 15, 194
workplace 28, 53–4, 259
World Bank 138, 140, 148, 149

World Health Organization (WHO) 138, 140
breastfeeding 147
co-ordinated action 260
definition of health 4, 32
essential drug list 144, 146
ethical targets 89
'Health for All' strategy 2, 30–1, 34–9, 145, 260
regional offices 148
World health reports 138, 141, 149

Name/Title Index

Aristotle (*Politics*) 231

Bacon, F. 114, 118
Banks, Sir J. 265
Beatson, Sir G. 108
Bernard, Saint 179
Brown, Dr. J. 181
Buber, M.
  I and thou 67, 86, 180

Callaghan, D.
  What kind of life 7, 29, 177, 264
Calman, K. 45, 104
  Healthy respect 45, 88, 96
  Hospital doctors: training for the future 211, 242
  Calman/Hine Report 213
Campbell, J.
  The hero with a thousand faces 183, 188
Carlyle, T. 129
Chekov, A.
  Ward 6 98
Clarke, B.
  Whose life is it anyway? 99
Clausewitz, C. von
  On war 21
Cronin, A.J 224
Crummy, H.
  Let the people sing 102
Cuthbertson, Sir D. 135

Dennison, A.
  An uncertain journey 99
Disraeli, B. 8
  Sybil 93, 96
Downie, R.S. 104, 230
  Health promotion 88, 96
  Healthy respect 45, 88, 96
Dunn, D.
  Elegies 100
Duthie, M. 104

Eliot, T.S. 178
  The cocktail party 99

Evans, R.J.
  Death in Hamburg 9, 29

Filde, Sir L. 224
Flexner, A. 103

Gairdner, Sir W.T. 117, 202
Galbraith, J.K.
  The good society 43, 45, 93, 96
Gardner, H.
  Leading minds 183, 188
Gillis, C. 210, 241
Gordon, R. 224
Griffiths, Sir R. 173

Hart, H.L.A.
  The concept of law 37, 45
Haward, R. 210, 241
Heberden, Dr. 202–3
Hippocrates 9, 197, 216–23, 263
Holmes, O.W.
  The professor at the breakfast table 153
Holmes, Sherlock 106, 113
Hunter, J. 202
Hunter, W. 202
Huxley, J. 30

Ibsen, H.
  Enemy of the people 99

Johnson, Dr. S. 153, 203

Kant, E. 61
Kelvin, Lord 114-15
King, M.L. 265
Kotter, J.
  The general manager 173
Kung, H.
  Global responsibility 93, 96, 264

Littlejohn, Sir H. 117

MacEwan, Sir W. 202
Mann, T.
  The magic mountain 99
Medawar, P. 115
Mooney, G. 128

Newman, Cardinal 29
Newman, Sir G. 202
Niklaus, J. 265

Osler, Sir W. 103, 202

Peters, R.S. 230

Rawls, J.
  A theory of justice 37, 45
Rowntree, S.
  Poverty: a study of town life 40, 45

Selby, D. 210, 241
Shakespeare, W. 167, 172, 192
Shaw, B.
  The doctor's dilemma 224
Smith, A. 265
  The wealth of nations 40
Stones, E.
  Psychology of education 262
Sweeney, B. 104
Sydenham, T. 202

Tannahill, D. & C.
  Health promotion 88, 96
Tauber, A.I. 104
Tournier, P.
  Creative suffering 68, 86, 182
Toynbee, A.J.
  A study of history 42
Twain, M. 158

Virchow, H. 172

Walker, M.E.M.
  Pioneers of health 114, 137
Welsh, I.
  Trainspotting 101